BETTER
THAN
BEAUTY

BY *Helen Valentine* & *Alice Thompson*

WITH ILLUSTRATIONS BY EMERY I. GONDOR

BETTER THAN BEAUTY

A Guide to Charm

CHRONICLE BOOKS
SAN FRANCISCO

ORIGINALLY PUBLISHED IN 1938 BY HERALD
PUBLISHING CO., NEW YORK, N.Y.

LIBRARY OF CONGRESS CATALOGING-IN-
PUBLICATION DATA:

Valentine, Helen. Better than beauty : a guide to charm / by
Helen Valentine and Alice Thompson ; with illustrations by
Emery I. Gondor.
p. cm.
Originally published: New York, N.Y. : Modern Age Books, 1938.
ISBN 0-8118-3451-4
1. Beauty, Personal. 2. Charm. I. Thompson,
Alice (Alice Dickey) II. Gondor, Emery I. III. Title.
RA778 .V25 2001   646.7'042—dc21   2001042368

Printed in the United States of America
Designed by Vivien Sung
Typeset by Blue Friday Type & Graphics

Distributed in Canada by Raincoast Books
9050 Shaughnessy Street
Vancouver, British Columbia V6P 6E5

10 9 8 7 6 5

CHRONICLE BOOKS LLC
85 SECOND STREET
SAN FRANCISCO, CALIFORNIA 94105
WWW.CHRONICLEBOOKS.COM

We dedicate this little book to two women
who undoubtedly could profit by reading it.

TO A. T. AND H. V.

Contents

BETTER THAN BEAUTY

A Guide to Charm

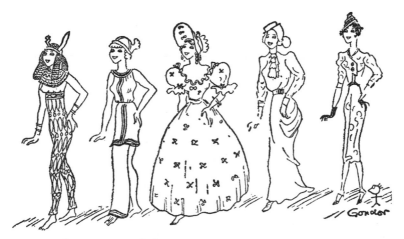

Every era has its concept of charm

Introduction

EVERY ERA has its own concept of charm. It springs from the current ways of life. The languorous woman had her place in the secure world of the eighteen nineties. The hoyden had her place in the shattered postwar epoch. Both were charming in so far as they blended with the scenery and needs of their period. In short, charm has many ageless qualities, but its outward signs are born of the period, the day's news, the tempo of the times. The charming woman, whether she slopped around in unbuckled galoshes, or drove part-time shifts in a prairie schooner, was the one who evaluated her epoch and accepted its standards, at least sufficiently to spare herself accidental bumps.

This restless time is so varied, so quick in its changes, that it takes a mental trapeze artist to discover and accept its framework. New social orders have come into being. New words describing new forms of government and new techniques have come into the language. Some of the very things we have come to accept as immutable are being scrutinized and hotly debated—freedom of speech, democracy, the right to eat, the pursuit of happiness, liberty versus authoritarianism. With such a rapidly shifting picture, the modern woman, as apt to be working as at home, has no easy task discovering what her role should be. Is it charming to be hard? Is it charming to question fundamentals? Is it even wise? Should one bother with charm in a troubled world?

Let's answer the last question first. No matter how wide your horizon, no matter how profound your convictions, you still function on a small piece of the canvas of our world. It is easier to live smoothly, to make your background recede into its proper place, if you live charmingly. It is easier to make your convictions acceptable to others, if you add charm to reason.

You should bother with charm in any sort of world, at home or in an office. The real problem is what constitutes charm for this particular era. And we are going to scratch down to the bare bones of some rather personal problems right now.

Part One:

WHAT YOU DO TO
YOURSELF

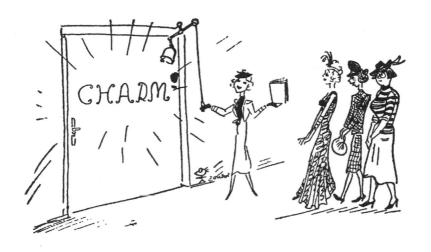

1 *Prelude to Charm*

ONCE in a lifetime you may meet that rare person whose face and appearance you forget, but whose charm remains indelible. It doesn't happen often. What we *see* usually becomes a vital part of our impression of people, our brain picture.

Your skin, your makeup, your hair, your hands, the way you sit, the way you stand—these are the priming coat, the background upon which all other qualities are imposed. What can you do to make your physical self more

7

expressive of that important inner quality of warmth and friendliness?

What your skin needs

If you get a great lift out of a dozen sweet-smelling jars of creams and lotions on your dressing table, buy all you can afford. But buy them for their morale-building qualities. There are only three things a normal skin needs. Abnormal skin needs a doctor.

Your skin needs a healthy diet. It can be no better than your stomach and your blood. Plenty of water, green vegetables, fruits, eggs, milk (but no excesses in food or drink) make your body healthy and are a basic diet for a healthy skin.

The second necessity is proper external cleansing. Twice a day your skin must be thoroughly cleansed. You may belong to the soap and water school or the cream-cleansing school. The surest technique, and one that will serve for all parts of the country, is the combination of cream and soap and water. You can use this in the very dry West, the very humid East, and the dusty in-betweens. Give your face and neck a thorough application of any good cream, a gentle but complete wiping off, and then a lathery face-wash with a mild soap and warm water, followed by a rinse with cool water. The very dry skin that peels easily may need a light coating of cream after the rinse.

The third essential is becoming makeup. And the clue is in the word "becoming." Your makeup must become a part of you. If it is so off-key, if it is so startling that it dazzles, or so underdone that it causes spectators to worry over your health, it is not part of you. Freakish eyebrows, gooey eyelids, too-pale cheeks, and completely untouched-by-beauty-aids faces are all unnatural. "What! No makeup at all unnatural?" For an urban woman under sixty, yes! For though that woman may be as nature made her, she will look colorless among her brightened-up sisters.

Makeup is a very simple matter of using your eyes, your color sense, and your hand. Any woman who can match a sample of thread to a piece of fabric can select the correct shades of makeup for herself. And any woman who can hold a pencil and make it write can apply lip-rouge, powder, and other cosmetics to her face. There is no magic, no mystery, no hidden trick.

Makeup routine

Here is the routine—a ten-minute task for an amateur, a three-minute performance for an old hand.

1. Your face is clean. Apply an all-over foundation cream (any reputable brand) in a shade that matches your skin tone.

2. With the light shining *on* your face, prepare to do the rest of the job. If this is a daytime makeup, take a mirror (you can get a very adequate one for thirty cents) to the window, hang it on the window lock, and face it.

3. Dip a big powder puff in a light-textured face powder that matches your skin tone; *pat* the powder on all over your face. Put on plenty.

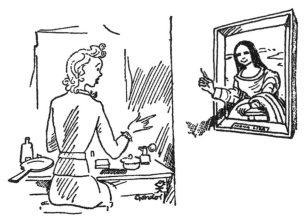

This isn't a mural for the Louvre . . .

4. Use a soft powder brush (they're sold in ten-cent stores) to brush off the excess powder.

5. Apply rouge lightly to the cheeks. Never mind all the confusing details of planes and angles. This isn't

a mural for the Louvre, it's your face. And you know, without art lessons, that natural color doesn't grow in splotchy circles or streaky lines or huge rose-pink areas. Put your rouge on so that it looks

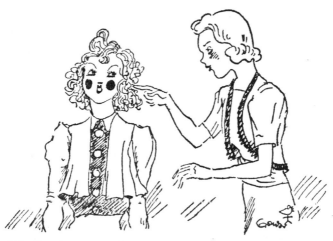

Color doesn't grow in splotchy circles

like your own color, and blend it with your powder so that it fades into the normal shade of your own skin.

6. Use a good quality lipstick. Again, use your color sense in choosing the shade of lipstick. If you are a white-skinned brunette with a faint blue cast to your skin, use a lipstick that tends toward the raspberry. If

you are creamy-skinned with more yellow in your skin, use a lipstick that verges on the orange shades. The major job in lipstick application, and the one most neglected, is the *completion* of the task. The casual smear, the quick once-over, will not work. Get that brutal light on your face and apply your lipstick meticulously, so that it covers all parts of the lips evenly. Now bite down on a piece of cleaning tissue. This takes off the excess and prevents that most unlovely accident—lipstick on your teeth.

7. If your brows are blonde or not well defined, use an eyebrow pencil lightly. And if you are out to be devastating, mascara on your eyelashes won't hinder you.

Once you are made up, forget it. You won't need powder or lipstick for at least three hours. And when you do need repairing, retire to a ladies' room, and repair carefully. The quick dab of powder and lipstick that we put on in public, we put on badly, probably because we don't want to seem too interested in the performance. And no matter how much acceptance-through-custom this may have, the public performance of private beauty rites is not attractive. It is permissible when there is no retiring room—at a football game, for instance.

Your hair

There is more old-wivery and hocus-pocus on the subject of hair than you could read in years. The first great question that comes up in any discussion is "How often should hair be washed?" The answer is the same for everyone whose hair and general health are normal. Hair, like any other part of your body, should be washed when it is dirty. And don't let this sentence start a mental argument about your dry scalp or your oily scalp. If you live in an industrial center where coal dust rules the waves, your hair needs laundering once or twice a week. If your scalp is too dry, oil it before the shampoo, and use a little brilliantine afterward. If it is too oily, omit this. And forget the theorizing.

The next points are the soap and the rinses. Any good soap that you would use on your body is correct for your hair. If the water in your vicinity is hard, melt your soap in water first, to make a liquid shampoo.

Lemon juice, vinegar, and all other grease-cutting rinses will help get the last remnants of soap from your hair. But they are not necessary if your water supply is unlimited.

Keep your hair clean between washings by brushing it regularly. Never mind the mythical hundred strokes. Just get it brushed thoroughly.

There can be no general diagnosis of the way all women should wear their hair. And yet, many a woman has missed loveliness by a poor coiffure. The best advice that can be given is to get rid of any preconceived ideas of your "type." Look in the mirror at a stranger. Look at her face as though you didn't know how she had ever worn her hair before. Start to experiment. You can do it yourself and have a good time in the process. Of course it is pleasant to

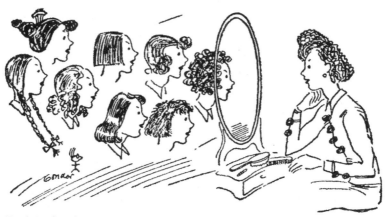

Look in the mirror at a stranger

go to the finest hairdresser in town and have him or her design and dress your hair. But even this won't make a change for the better until you get away from ideas about how you can and can't wear your hair. If you do go to a professional, insist upon only one thing. Make sure the coiffure is one you can at least approximate in your own boudoir.

Last, but far from least, remember that hair must look like itself to be pleasant. The lacquered, the extreme, the "artificial color added," are not lovely. Your surest guide is a simple one. Does your hair look as though it would be pleasant to touch—clean, fresh, alive, soft?

Hands tell tales

Charming hands need not be perfect hands. Advertisements to the contrary, people do not stare at your hands unless you force that attention. And so the goal to be reached is not perfection. We can't change the shape of our fingers and palms, but we can do a lot with their appearance.

Cleanliness comes first. Does that seem almost insultingly obvious? But stop. Think how often your hands get a quick washing, leaving the ground-in dirt still lodged in the lines of the skin. Your wash basin may need equipment. It should have a good soap, a good brush, a mild but thorough grease solvent, an orange stick, and a goodly bottle of hand lotion. After you have scrubbed out the dirt, use the orange stick. This process belongs with washing. Now the hand lotion. The brand matters very little, but faithful application matters much.

Keep another large bottle of hand lotion in the kitchen. You notice we emphasize the hand lotion as a part of cleanliness. It is. Rough hands become dirty far more quickly than smooth ones.

Rubber gloves are worth the time and effort spent in caring for them, if you do much housework. When you are tempted to think they make you awkward, remember that a surgeon does his most delicate work with rubber-gloved hands.

After your hands are clean and smooth, there are the nails to be cared for. They are a nuisance. Manicuring is a picky job. But unmanicured hands are much more of a nuisance. You're always thinking about them, vaguely, and vainly trying to keep them out of sight.

The manicure need not be a ritual. It has only three aims: to keep the cuticle under control, to add color or luster to your nails, and to keep the nails the right length. Your occupation determines that length. The typist who affects long nails gets chipped and broken ones. Ditto the saleswoman or the busy housewife. In general it is best to keep your nails only slightly longer than the pads of your fingertips.

You need set aside no one time to do all three manicuring tasks. When your nails need filing, it is logical to shape them as you file. The cuticle is something that should be given a little prod every time you dry your hands. Just push it back gently with the towel while it is soft. And put some oil or lanolin on it in the evenings before bedtime, if it seems to get ragged. The polishing can't be run according to one schedule for all women. Mrs. Robertson puts her brilliant liquid polish on once a week, and there it stays unchipped, untarnished, and perfect. Mrs. Ainsworth, who has a small baby and must have her hands in water frequently, needs fresh polish every other day. Only you can know how often your nails need polish—but bear in mind that nothing is more conspicuous than chipped, cracked fingernail polish. Better none at all.

We said hands tell tales. Be sure yours tell the best of the truth. There is nothing unpleasant about hands that look as though they did housework—nothing unpleasant while they are doing the housework. But just as you change your housedress when you go out, so you should keep your hands in a state that will permit them to change their garb, too. Prematurely dried-out, thick-skinned hands are ugly, and unnecessary when even inexpensive salad oil will serve as lotion.

Start looking at other people's hands and analyze what you find pleasant and unpleasant. You will probably bar the claw-fingernails. You should. The overlong fingernail is predatory, unpleasant.

The color of your polish is an individual matter. Well-shaped hands and nails can take brilliant tones. All others should be made as inconspicuous as possible. Bright red pulls the eyes to the hands. Be sure yours can stand those eyes before you use the attention getter.

The last thing to remember about hands is that though they stop at the wrists, the eye of the beholder does not. The very measures you take to keep your hands clean and soft should be carried up the wrists, with a special second or so spent on the elbows.

Your feet are your fortune

Feet and popularity are close relations. If you don't believe it, remember the dance when you had a painful corn; the tea when your shoes pinched; the hike with a gay companion, when there was a blister on your heel; the dinner party when the satin slippers began to cut across your instep.

Your face can't look serene, your conversation can't be bright, your personality can't radiate, if your feet hurt. The worst of it is that the hurt need not be acute. Even the most minor foot discomfort can erase charm and add years.

Yet there's nothing complicated about the proper care of the feet. A weekly clipping of toenails, a scrupulous cleanliness, stockings that are long enough but not too long, shoes fitted by an expert, are all that is necessary. With these simple measures, normal feet will stay at the bottom of your body instead of leaving their prints on your face and feelings.

If your feet are not normal, go to a doctor and start right in to restore their health. But the usual ills that beset our feet do not need a doctor. They need only common sense and two general types of good shoes. The shoes you

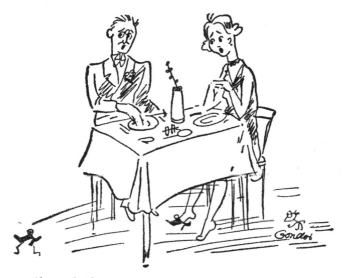

. . . if your feet hurt

use for every day and walking need not look like orthopedic models. Comfort does indicate lower heels and real support in these shoes, however. Your afternoon shoes should be more flattering. Of course they should fit you perfectly, but they can have a higher heel and be styled for beauty rather than practicality.

Your carriage, madame!

When we think of women who stand and walk and sit with distinction, our minds visualize the late eighteen nineties and early nineteen hundreds. They certainly stood up and sat straight, those ironclad, corseted-to-the-chin mothers and grandmothers of ours. But rigid ramrods are out of date. None of us is going back to that painfully restricted era. Neither have we hours to spend walking with books on our heads, nor the leisure to practice how to sit down gracefully.

Rigidity is not necessary when you are aiming at good posture. It isn't even a good goal. But most of us have at least one ugly and easily changed fault of carriage.

Are you the toilworn type, the woman who walks with bent shoulders and drooped middle? Get rid of the mental attitude, tuck in your stomach, and watch your body straighten! Are you the inquiring duck-neck, carrying your head about three inches ahead of your body? Back up against a wall and make your head touch the wall, too. Get the feel of this proper position, and check yourself as you pass reflecting windows and mirrors.

Do you toe out in the genteel, outmoded fashion of 1912? Make a conscious effort to get those toes straight ahead. Have you the arrogant bustle walk, your hips thrown out behind? Start today, learning to walk as though someone were about to spank you—and watch those hips go back where they came from.

Your walk should be distinguished by its lack of outstanding qualities. You don't want people to notice your

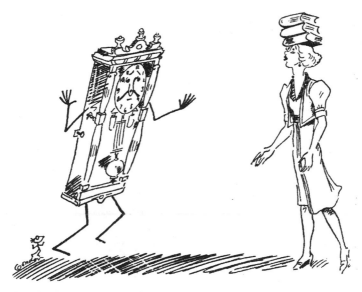

Neither have we hours to spend . . .

posture, good or bad. You want them to see you. So correct the faults that attract attention and forget the rest.

Much the same rule applies to sitting. No one will wait to watch how gracefully you lower yourself into a chair.

No one cares. But if you drop in a manner to frighten the owner of the chair, you will get plenty of attention. And if you insist on sitting either like a disapproving maiden aunt or a licentious Roman diner, people will notice you, too. But it won't be your charm they notice. The most prevalent and the ugliest of all sitting-faults is the frog-leg squat—and squat is the only word. You know

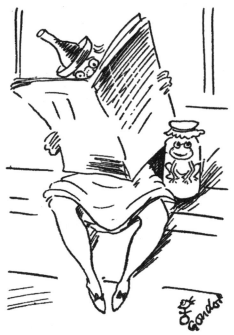

. . . the frog-leg squat

it. The feet are either together or apart, but the legs are widespread at the knees.

Learn to walk and sit in an apparently effortless, graceful manner. Then you can be sure you will have learned to carry yourself well.

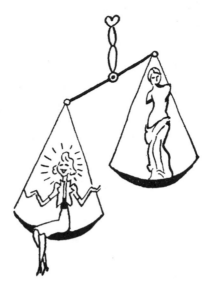

2   *Your Best Friends*

YOUR mirror, your scales, your nose—these, frankly, are your best friends. On them you can depend for an honest picture and for unbiased criticism.

No woman with any claim to charm would ever wait for any other "best friend" to tell her that she has put on too much weight or has an unpleasant body odor. The latter especially is one of the things you must recognize instantly and correct immediately. It is death on charm. It can alienate friends faster than the most charming woman can acquire them!

But to attend to friend number one, your scales. It is undoubtedly a good idea to watch your weight. You needn't make a fetish of it, but every week or so check up on yourself. Don't be the sort of person who is constantly talking about her weight: "I'm so pleased. I've lost two pounds this week and I'm back to my 122," or "I don't know what's the matter with me, I've watched my diet, but I can tell by my clothes that I've been putting on weight again."

These matters are your affair. They are of interest to you, but they are of scant importance to everyone else.

What should you weigh?

This is a question on which tomes have been written. But it boils down to a few simple points. If you are a great deal overweight or a great deal underweight, by all means consult a doctor. Abnormal weight may be a symptom of some other disturbance, not necessarily serious, but certainly worth taking care of.

If you are slightly overweight or underweight you can try remedying the condition yourself, sensibly, with not too drastic changes in your diet or your living plan. But, even then, it is better to consult a physician first.

Before you consider your weight remember that, in general, it is well for a woman under thirty to be slightly overweight. During these early years the body still can use this extra defense against disease. After thirty, it is far better to be slightly underweight. That lessens the strain on the heart and on other organs, and gives a better chance for health and longer life.

Think of all the very old people you ever knew. Can you recall any who was fat? Usually, the people who reach a ripe old age are exceedingly thin, and they grow thinner as they grow older. Too much fat may be a menace to health as well as to charm. So be sensible, and do something about it. Here is a table of average weights for women.

AVERAGE WEIGHT ACCORDING TO HEIGHT AND AGE

This table is based on the Medico-Actuarial study of more than 130,000 insured women.*

Height (with shoes) Feet Inches	Weight in Pounds According to Age (as ordinarily dressed)								
	15 to 19	20 to 24	25 to 29	30 to 34	35 to 39	40 to 44	45 to 49	50 to 54	55 to 59
5 1	112	117	120	123	126	130	133	135	137
5 2	115	120	122	125	129	133	136	138	140
5 3	118	123	125	128	132	136	139	141	143
5 4	121	126	129	132	136	139	142	144	146
5 5	124	129	132	136	140	143	146	148	150
5 6	128	133	136	140	144	147	151	152	153
5 7	132	137	140	144	148	151	155	157	158
5 8	136	141	144	148	152	155	159	162	163
5 9	140	145	148	152	156	159	163	166	167
5 10	144	149	152	155	159	162	166	170	173

*These figures are reproduced by courtesy of The Metropolitan Life Insurance Company. Their table carries this important legend—"The Average Weight Is Not Always the Best Weight."

In other words, women with large frames may weigh a bit more without looking fat. Women with tiny frames cannot afford too many extra pounds. So, be guided by the way you feel and the way you look. When clothes no longer seem becoming, that is a sure signal to start doing something about your figure.

If you are too fat

Granted you need to lose some extra poundage. How do you start? By a visit to a doctor, to be sure that moderate dieting and exercise will not be harmful. By planning a healthful weight-reducing diet and sticking to it. By planning a set of exercises and doing them consistently. By keeping your bowels open.

You should *not* take reducing tablets or medicines, however tempting their advertising may be. Any drug that is potent enough to reduce you, may also be harmful. No drug of this type should ever be taken except upon the advice of a physician.

You should not lose more than two pounds a week. Even a pound and a half is enough. Do your losing slowly and steadily. Do not be discouraged if, after a week or two of dieting, you have not lost at all. Continue with your routine. You will soon be rewarded.

A safe reducing diet contains about 1500 calories a day. In the back of the book there is a list showing the caloric content of several hundred foods. From it you can learn just which foods to avoid.

Once you've learned that one macaroon has as many calories as a large head of lettuce, or that one chocolate

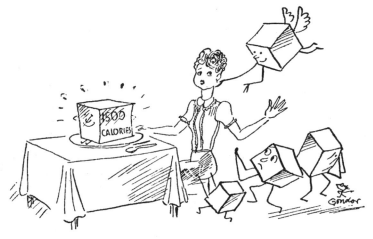

1500 calories a day

soda equals sixteen cups of consommé, or that two tablespoons of cream have more calories than half a grapefruit, you'll think before you eat. You will learn to plan meals that have plenty of variety and nutrition, but not too many calories.

It can be done. And remember that alcohol has a high number of calories, so be sure to count it in with your food.

Avoid those dieting blues

To diet intelligently, you should know which foods the body needs for health, and which add the extra fat.

Every body needs food for fuel to keep it going through its usual activities. In addition, it needs a little extra to repair the daily wear and tear.

A normal diet should have protein (meat, fish, eggs, etc.), fats (butter, cream, fat meats, etc.), carbohydrates (potatoes, bread, pastry, etc.), salt (contained in certain fruits and vegetables), vitamins, and water.

A badly balanced reducing diet can be definitely harmful. And, even when it is not actually so, it can make you feel miserable. Nothing is as unattractive as a woman with the dieting blues. She is irritable, jumpy. She sacrifices any physical advantage of lost weight, when she also loses her temper. Watch yourself, lady—as well as your scales.

Which foods are fattening?

The most fattening foods are: cream soups, fried meats, fried potatoes, cheeses, cream, butter, oil, puddings, pies, pastries, candy, ice cream, chocolate, cocoa.

Good foods for a reducing diet are: clear soups or beef broth, fish (particularly flounder and cod), lean meats,

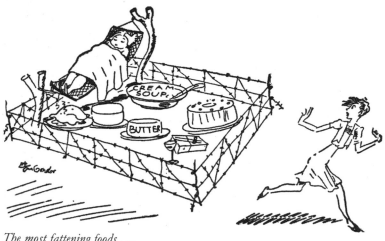

The most fattening foods . . .

especially beef, lamb, chicken, ham. Almost all fruits, but especially the following: apples, apricots, berries (without sugar and cream, of course), cantaloupe, oranges, peaches, grapefruit, pineapple, pears, watermelon, lemons.

You need all kinds of vegetables, but eat sparingly of the starchy ones like potatoes and corn and peas. Best are string beans, tomatoes, asparagus, beets, cabbage, rhubarb, cauliflower, lettuce, endive, watercress, spinach, artichokes, broccoli, eggplant, sauerkraut, Brussels sprouts, celery, cucumbers, leeks, radishes, squash, turnips, carrots, onions.

Tea and coffee (without cream or sugar), eggs, butter-milk, cottage cheese, and skimmed milk may be in your "can eat" list.

But are you muttering, "It's all very well to talk about certain foods, but I have to plan meals for a family, not just for myself. My children need plenty of fattening foods. How can I have the right diet for them and for me at the same time?"

It's easy. For instance, if you have a roast meat for dinner, eat the meat but not the gravy or the fat. Take a slightly larger portion of the green vegetable and a very small helping of potatoes. If the dessert is fruit, eat it. If it's a pie or pudding, pass it by. Have a raw apple instead. But don't talk about your self-control and sacrifice.

But perhaps you're too thin

Since most women seem to worry about being over-weight, the thin woman's problems are often forgotten. But scrawniness isn't any more attractive or healthy than fatness. So try to cover the bones by eating the foods on our fattening list. Learn the luxury of extra meals, the mid-morning and mid-afternoon glass of milk with bread and butter, or crackers and jam, the easily digested snack, with a cup of cocoa just before you go to bed. Rest after your three main meals, if you can arrange it. Don't smoke too much. And don't fret about unimportant things, one of which is your weight.

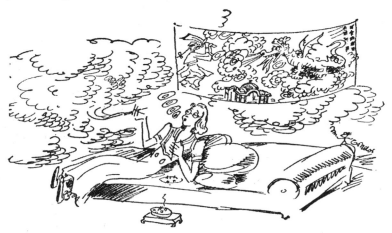

Don't smoke too much

Do you exercise?

If you do housework, the chances are you get plenty of exercise, though not necessarily balanced exercise. If you do little or no housework, or spend your days at an office desk, you certainly need a good exercise schedule. There's no use planning elaborate routines, because the odds are against your sticking to them. So make them few and simple, but do them every day. Morning or evening, or both, if you're serious.

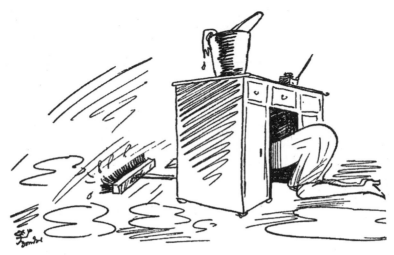

If you do housework . . .

Hip, hip . . . away!

One of the most common figure-faults seems to be weight at the hips, buttocks, and thighs—a sort of general below-the-waistline heaviness. These exercises are designed to attack this problem, and reduce it by several inches.

Exercise 1—This is our old friend, Rolling. Sit on the floor with legs straight and feet together. Put your hands on the floor; a little behind you and out to the sides.

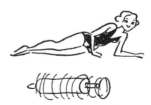

Roll over to the left while you lift your right hand and put it over by your left hand. Keep your elbows straight and stay in this position while you stretch and tense your muscles. Raise your head until you can see the backs of your knees. Relax and roll over to the other side. Repeat this six times the first day, working up until you can do it twenty times, without undue fatigue. Add two or three rolls each day.

Exercise 2—Lie on the floor with your feet together and your hands under the fattest part of your hips. Raise

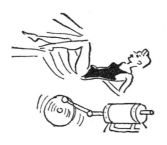

your right leg, bend your knee and draw it close to your body, straighten the leg and lower it to the floor. Do the same with your left leg. Then do both legs together. Do this six times the first day and work up to fifteen.

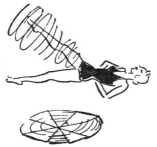

Exercise 3—Start in same position as Exercise 2. Raise your right leg a little and rotate it in as wide a circle as you can. Keep the leg straight. Do it first in one direction and then reverse and do it

backwards. Then rotate the other leg in the same way. Then hold both legs close together and rotate them at the same time. Start with six and work up to twelve. If you have difficulty keeping your shoulders down, let someone hold them for you until you gain sufficient control to do the exercise unaided.

Exercise 4—This is the famous Scissors. You lie on the floor on your left side, with your left arm under your head, stretched out, palm to the ceiling. Put your right hand on 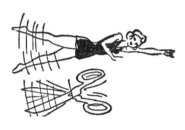 the floor in front of your chest. Lift both feet off the floor and move your legs back and forth as though you were walking. The movement must be in the hips and your knees must not bend. Your head and arms should be relaxed. Start with ten and work up to twenty.

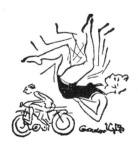 *Exercise 5*—This is the Bicycle. Lie on your back in the same position as Exercise 2. Raise both legs in the air, bend the knees and pedal the legs as though you were on a bicycle. Do this from ten to thirty times or

more. It is not a difficult exercise and will not tire you, even if you do it more than the other exercises.

These five, done regularly, should begin to show some result after about ten days. There are plenty of other good exercises, but if we give too many, will you do them all? Once you've formed the habit, you may want to add a few exercises to your original five.

No spare tires, please!

Clothes never look well on a figure that has too much flesh around the waistline or a flabby abdomen. If either or both of them is your problem, set to work on these:

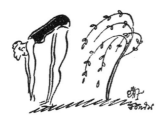

Exercise 1—Our old friend, Touching the Toes. Stand with your feet together, raise your arms high above your head and bend forward till your fingertips reach down toward your toes. If, at first, you cannot reach them with your knees rigid, bend your knees a little. Do not strain or stretch too hard. Relax at all times. Gradually you will be able to reach farther and farther. Eventually you will be able to do the exercise without bending your knees. Start with six bends. Add one each day until you work up to fifteen.

Exercise 2—Stand with your feet
fairly well apart and your arms over
your head. Lock your thumbs to
insure keeping your hands together.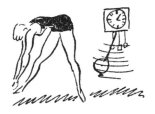
Twist your body to the right, bend
and touch the floor beyond your
right foot with both hands. Bend your right knee while you
do it. Raise your arms overhead, twist your trunk all the
way to the left and touch the floor outside your left foot,
bending your left knee. This exercise should be done in
one continuous flow of motion, without stopping. Start
with six the first day and work up to twenty, if you can. If
you find it too tiring, stop at fifteen.

Exercise 3—Stand with your
feet apart and your arms over
your head. Hold your arms against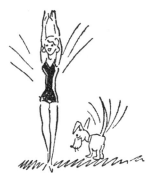
your ears, and lock your thumbs.
Then, keeping your hips still, bend
the top of your body from side to
side. Go as far as you can without
straining. Then lock your hands
behind your head and bend the
trunk forward and back. Start with six each and work up
to twenty.

Exercise 4—This one looks very easy, but it needs careful doing. Stand with your legs apart and arms stretched out at both sides, at right angles to your body. Then, holding your hips still, rotate your trunk. That is, bring your right arm and shoulder forward while your left go back, and vice versa. Watch two things in this exercise. Your arms

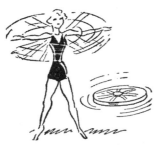

and shoulders must remain in the same relative positions *and* your hips must be kept still. It is a help to have someone actually hold your hips when you first do the exercise. Start with six, work up to twenty.

Exercise 5—Lie down on the floor with your arms above your head, your legs straight and your feet together. In one smooth motion raise your arms and body and bend forward until your hands touch your toes— or as close to your toes as you can. Then go back and repeat. Start with six and work up to fifteen.

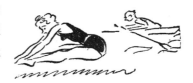

Incidentally, all the exercises given here provide a health-building routine for *anyone.* They will improve muscle tone and posture, they will help to correct faulty elimination, and they will give you a feeling of vigor and well being.

Have you wondered why the screen stars are blessed with such good figures? Don't attribute it to a gift from the kindly fates. Many of those stars have to wage a continual battle against weight. They exercise regularly, eat carefully, and live simply. They do the very things you should do. They lose their jobs if they don't. What you lose is attractiveness.

What do we mean by "clean"?

There isn't a woman of your acquaintance who wouldn't resent it if you accused her of being physically dirty. Yet, frankly, too few women are entirely clean.

There is Miss R. who wouldn't skip her morning bath if the skies fell. But I went with her one day when she was buying a dress. Her slip had grayish shoulder straps.

Then there's Mrs. K. who doubtless bathes with fair regularity but who is very hit-or-miss about the use of deodorants.

Miss B. still subscribes to that old wives' tale that it's bad for hair to wash it too often. So there is frequently a musty odor when you get too close to her.

Mrs. Q. changes her underthings often enough and abides by all rules of cleanliness, except—one is often reminded that Mrs. Q. has feet. A little personal spying on herself would tell her what others know. She needs a deodorant foot powder.

Miss T. keeps her face beautifully clean and correctly made up, but her fingernails are often dirty; her knuckles sometimes have that grimy, small-boy look.

These women are legion. They're nice people, too. How they would hate to be told that they aren't fastidious!

The only ways to play safe are to take a bath every day, change your underwear not less than every other day, change hosiery every day, use deodorants regularly. And . . .

Use your nose

Your most valuable best friend is your nose. By all means use it.

The advertising of deodorants and antiperspirants has certainly been painting a dramatic picture of lives ruined by body odors. Smile if you will, consider it exaggerated, but admit that there is a hard kernel of truth under it all.

Whether consciously or unconsciously, most people respond to pleasant smells and are repelled by unpleasant ones. One can't help wondering how often phrases like "a chemical attraction between people" and "I don't know why I dislike her, but I do" may have their true explanation in a sense of smell.

Do not confuse deodorants and antiperspirants. They are entirely different; but each has its place in the life of every fastidious human being.

Antiperspirants actually stop or deter perspiration. Deodorants neutralize perspiration and other body odors.

There are several good antiperspirants on the market. But equally effective and absolutely safe is a solution of Aluminum Chloride which any druggist can make up for you. A 15 percent solution is usually right for the average person. If you perspire excessively, you can have it made 20 or even 25 percent, but not stronger than that. Use it in your armpits after bathing. Just pat it on with a little pad of absorbent cotton. After it is dry, rinse it off with cool water. How often do you need an antiperspirant? Some people need it only once a week, some twice, some every day. Only you can tell.

Do not be afraid to stop underarm perspiration. The rest of your body still perspires, to a less intense degree, and adequately performs the function of ridding the body of certain waste. If, for any reason, you do not use a anti-perspirant, be sure that all your frocks are equipped with dress shields—and that these are always kept scrupulously clean and fresh. With these, you must use a deodorant.

Deodorants are available in powder and paste form. Both are effective. Use a deodorant whenever you suspect that you might be under any special emotional or physical strain. Nervous intensity often makes glands more active and therefore increases perspiration. And always use a deodorant on sanitary pads.

Another way in which your nose can serve you well is in warning you when certain dresses or blouses need a trip to the cleaner. Sometimes a dark dress may look fresh, but unless its underarm and across-the-back sections *smell* fresh, too, it should not be worn until it has been cleaned.

Friend number three—your mirror

Your full-length mirror is a friend indeed, if you will listen to what it tells you. Don't look into it just to find whether your hair is neat or your lipstick is on right. Study your mirror to find out about your posture.

Chapter 1, Page 20 told you a few important facts about posture. Study your mirror to see if your skirt hangs well, your hat is in the right proportion. Study it to see that you are well put together and carefully groomed. (Much more about this is coming in Chapter 3.)

Teeth for life

We know one woman whose only claim to beauty is her teeth. We know several women who would be beauties if it weren't for their teeth. But who knows anyone who likes going to the dentist?

Still, your teeth were planned to be a permanent fixture. As such, they deserve extra special care. Your hair grows out and changes, your skin is constantly being renewed. But your teeth are there for good.

Of course, care should start in infancy. But one can't retrace the years and correct sins of omission or commission. So, suppose your teeth aren't all they should be, what can you do?

Have a good dentist. If you cannot afford an expensive dentist, try to find a promising young man whose prices are still moderate, but whose skill is unquestionable. Perhaps your physician can help you find one. Or, if any private dentist is beyond your means, go to a good dental clinic.

The important thing is to go regularly. For a cleaning go at least twice a year, more often if you can afford it. That actually serves to catch dental troubles when they are just beginning. Since they are easiest and cheapest to correct then, frequent visits are an economy.

Your own care of your teeth should be a sacred rite. It is more important than any mere beauty culture, for it influences health as well as appearance.

Three times daily is the minimum number of times you should brush your teeth. Clean them when you get up, after breakfast, and at night just before going to bed. Always use a firm brush and either a good paste or powder.

After eating, it is well to brush your teeth just with water. That loosens food particles. It is an excellent habit. Need we mention that dental floss is a "must"?

We suggest that you have two toothbrushes, so that one is always dry and firm. Brushing your teeth with a wet soggy brush does them little good. Incidentally, the brushes last much longer if you give them a chance to dry thoroughly between usings.

Here's how!

When you drink, where you drink, how much you drink, whether you drink at all—these are most assuredly your own affair. Drinking and its relation to charm is discussed quite fully in Chapter 6. But just a word about drinking in relation to your appearance.

There are a few, a very few women, who can drink without having it show in their faces. But most women, if they drink more than a little, begin to acquire a telltale look. Their eyes are slightly duller, skin slightly sallower, lines slightly harder. Not a great change, of course, but a subtle one that is sensed rather than seen. It is an unattractive and disturbing change. At the first shadowy trace of it, the woman who cares about her appearance reduces her drinking to a veritable minimum. If she misses its stimulating effect and feels a letdown, she takes some added exercise, uses her brains to tackle an intricate problem, becomes

interested in something other than herself. She soon wonders why she ever needed liquor at all. And it isn't long
before her mirror tells a pleasanter tale.

Eight hours' sleep?

One of the hangovers from our childhood is the myth
about everyone needing eight hours of sleep. During our
years of growth, yes. But once you've reached the ripe old
age of twenty-four or twenty-five, stop worrying too much
about the amount of sleep you get.

Nature seems to know best. Some people need a lot of
sleep, some need a little. The main thing is to get as much
benefit as possible out of the hours you allot for sleeping.

If you wake up during the night, don't toss frantically
from side to side thinking "I'll be dead tired in the morning." Remember that lying quietly in bed is restful. It does
almost as much for a weary body as sleep. Relax and try to
keep your mind as blank as possible. And the chances are
you'll be drifting off to sleep before you know it.

Don't be the woman who regales her friends with:
"What a night I had! I went to bed at eleven and slept till
two. Then I woke up and I never closed my eyes again until
after the milkman had delivered the milk. What a night!"

Undoubtedly her night was not pleasant. But it
becomes definitely boring in the telling. If you have continual insomnia, by all means ask your physician about

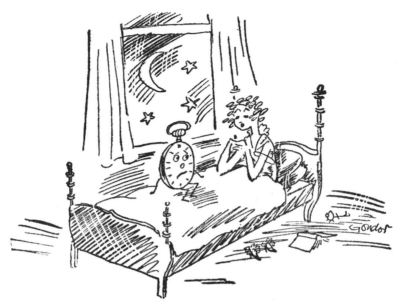

If you wake up during the night . . .

it. He may recommend a nonhabit-forming sedative for you. Taking one will do you far less harm than worrying about your lack of sleep.

"She walks in beauty"

Lord Byron doubtless had a poetic vision of some rare and exquisite creature when he wrote that beautiful phrase. But to a modern world, walking in beauty is something which every woman can achieve. She goes forth . . . rested, clean,

carefully groomed . . . she wears comfortable and becoming
clothes . . . she carries her head up, her shoulders back . . .
she exudes an aura of quiet assurance. She does, indeed,
walk in beauty.

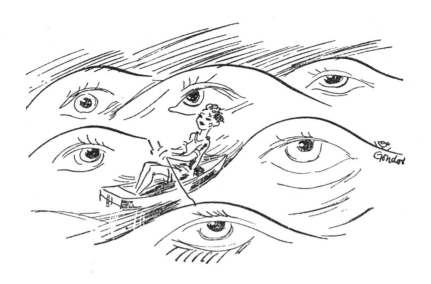

3 The Visual Side of Charm

OUR world has placed such a premium on chic that few women can be truly charming about it. You may like it or not; the fact remains.

When is a woman chic?

Just what do we mean when we say a woman looks chic? That she is dressed to the hilt? That she looks as though she spent her life at the dressmaker's? That she is carefully coifed with never a hair out of place? Not by any means! Chic must not appear studied. It must look as though it had just happened. Spend as much time as you need to in front of your mirror, but never, never look as though you had!

Glance at the word itself. "Chic" is a French word which we have taken over because we have never found its equivalent in our own language. Fashion magazines have tried for years to find a substitute for this much-used monosyllable. They've even offered prizes for a suitable English version, but without success. What do we mean, what do the French mean, when they say "chic"?

A woman who dresses well? Yes, and a great deal more. A woman who knows her type and intensifies it; a woman who wears clothes that dramatize her good points and conceal her faults; a woman who is never overdressed and never too conscious of her clothes. Yes, all of these, but even more—a woman with a certain verve and spirit and dash. Yes, a woman with charm! For chic is certainly the visual aspect of charm.

Optical illusions

You are a certain type of person and want to know how to improve your appearance. We'll take various kinds of figures and see what can be done for them. But first, let us show you one very simple trick. You've probably seen it before. But study it again to see how lines can create illusions.

Which of these lines is longer? Which of these women is taller? You guess. Well, which is? They're both the same,

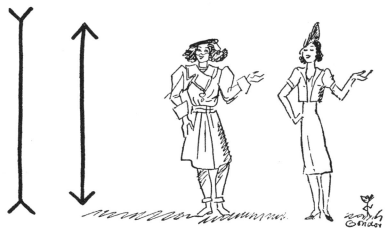

Which of these women is taller?

as you will see if you measure. But the placing of those little arrows makes a mighty difference. Mere lines can create illusions. Your clothes can make you look taller or shorter, thinner or rounder, just as you wish.

If you are very short

With fashion figures a good six feet tall and mannequins long and slender, it is sometimes easy for a short woman to develop a slight feeling of inferiority about her appearance. That's nonsense. Men like small women. But the trick, when you're small, is to keep everything in scale. Develop your sense of proportion. Do not carry enormous handbags or wear overpowering pieces of jewelry. Do not wear large hats—they make a small girl look like an umbrella. Do not wear wide belts or flowing sashes. Keep everything in scale.

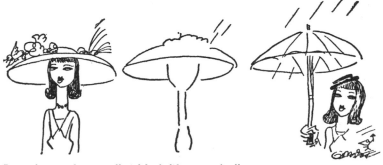

Large hats make a small girl look like an umbrella

It is important to watch your weight. A tall woman can get away with a few added pounds, but you can't. Keep slim. That helps create an illusion of height. Watch your carriage. Your head should always be held erect, your shoulders back. A slouch can steal inches.

What kind of clothes should you choose? Simple ones, naturally. Cut off the doo-dads; you can't afford them. You know that lines that go crosswise will cut you off, so try always to find clothes that have definite up-and-down lines. Choose long coats, rather than short, boxy ones; fitted coats, rather than very flared ones. Avoid large, bulky fur collars and fox neckpieces. If you have a fur collar, be sure it is small and of a flat fur. Or choose a collarless coat and wear a smallish scarf of wool or silk or fur, depending on the season and the amount of money you want to spend.

When you wear prints, be sure to choose the small ones, tiny dots or flowers, preferably regularly spaced. Avoid large, splashy patterns and too-vivid colors.

Do not wear your skirts too short. An extra half inch on your skirt adds height. And keep your belts at the natural waistline or above. If you are slender and Princess lines are in fashion, you can wear them well. But when you wear a belt, be sure it is narrow, and not too conspicuous. The too-noticeable belt can cut you in half in a distressing manner.

Some short women think they can improve their appearance by teetering around on extra-high heels. Not so. They are perfect for eveningwear, but on the street it is far smarter to wear average-height walking heels. And if you choose very simple shoes, preferably without straps, your legs will look longer.

Tiny hats, berets, and turbans are fine for you. You can wear a brim, if it is not too wide. But never buy a hat while you are seated in front of a mirror. Always stand up and study your full length. If the hat seems over-important, don't buy it.

Don't wear your hair too long and fluffy. It will make your head look disproportionate, giving the same effect as an overlarge hat. A sleek coiffure is far better for you.

Your most instinctive fashion horror should be *fussiness*. Omit all the extras. If there is any accessory you can leave off, by all means do so. If you would be truly charming, avoid cuteness in clothes and manner. And never talk baby talk.

If you are very tall

If you are very tall and thin, sing glory hallelujah. These days there's really no such thing as being *too* tall and thin. Most women would probably give their eyeteeth to have your figure. But it is important for you to know how to dress. If you are very slim, the chances are that you have bony shoulders and a prominent collarbone. But,

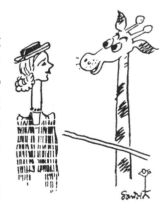

It is important to know how to dress

of all the faults the human figure is heir to, these are the easiest to conceal. High necklines are smart and promise to continue to be so for some time. But even when they are out, there is a type of high, wide, batteau line that has a classic and undying chic. Wear it, by all means. And wear broad shoulders (not exaggerated, sticking-out fancy-business, but genuine width) and generous scarfs around your neck. Accentuate your slim waist by exaggerating the bulk above. Wide belts and sashes are perfect on you, and on practically no one else.

Not for you a rigidly narrow silhouette, no matter how much in fashion it may be. It will make you look like the proverbial string bean. Always be sure that one part of your body is considerably wider than the rest. Preferably let it be your shoulders. The ideal silhouette for you has broad shoulders, pinched-in waist (at the normal waistline), and a slender, not-too-full skirt. Always try to adapt the prevailing mode to approximate these lines as closely as you can.

Your jewelry should be large and important looking. Heavy gold or silver chains with or without semiprecious stones, wide bracelets, large rings. Not too many at a time, please. Do not wear any dinky little jewels, however precious they may be. Several strands of pearls will always be more becoming to you than a single string. And don't forget that you are one of the few who can smartly carry a very large handbag.

Never have your clothes too tightly fitted. Casually fitted and draped lines are far better. Bulky furs, which engulf your smaller sister, make you look regal and

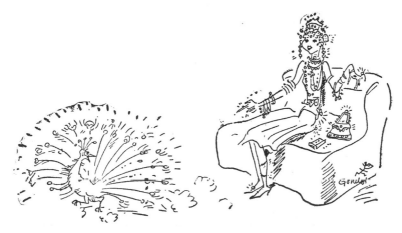

. . . not too many at a time, please

dramatic. Large hats, which make a small girl look out of balance, make you look romantic and interesting.

Your hair should not be cut too short. Always wear it long enough to avoid that unattractive pinhead look which very tall women sometimes inflict upon themselves.

What kind of shoes? Your first tendency will doubtless be to choose very low heels because you think they will detract from your height. But, unless you have the sort of feet and ankles and the manner of walking that can get away with flat heels, do not wear them. What you lose in height you also lose in grace. Wear the heels that look best on you, regardless of their height. Never be afraid of an extra half-inch.

That brings us to the matter of your posture. Slouching will not make you look shorter, it will merely make you look ungainly and awkward. Carry yourself as though you were proud of your height, as well you may be!

In the evening, avoid dresses with narrow shoulder straps and too-clinging fabrics. When prints are good, let yourself go on the splashy, dramatic variety that so few people can get away with.

Wear sports clothes whenever you can, bulky topcoats and tweedy suits and sweaters. Just be sure your sweater isn't tight. But a loose sweater and a generous scarf are quite perfect.

Woolens, heavy crêpes, and heavy cottons will doubt-less look better on you than thin materials, except when you choose chiffon, which can be graceful. Fabrics that cling too closely reveal bony parts. Fabrics with bulk (not necessarily stiffness) are better.

If you are too thin, try to put on a few pounds. But if you are well covered, consider your height a gift from the gods.

If you are stout

If you are stout, you can do one of two things. You can lose weight or you can make the best of the figure you have. If you want to do the former, see Chapter 2. For the latter, read on.

Haven't you seen plenty of stout women who wear very tight clothes? They look as though they had been forced into a sausage skin. Nothing accentuates fat so much as too-tight clothing. This is true in the fit of all parts of your dress, true of the sleeves, true even of your corset. That held-in look is not fashionable and certainly not slenderizing. Since all clothes look wrong on a too-rigid foundation, the large woman must go to a reliable *corsetière*.

Instead of trying to subtract inches by compressing yourself, use the optical illusion trick on page 50. Use it to best advantage by studying the lines of everything you buy. Never choose anything because it is "pretty," or a "sweet color," or "just like the one Marjorie has." Be sure it is right for *you* before you think of investing a single dollar.

Let's start with your dress. Every up-and-down line helps your figure, every horizontal line will hurt it. That's the first fundamental. Never lose sight of it. Don't succumb to dresses that have complicated lines or trimmings. Keep to the simple, flowing, vertical lines always. Your most becoming neckline will doubtless be a V. This will give your neck a longer look. A slightly draped

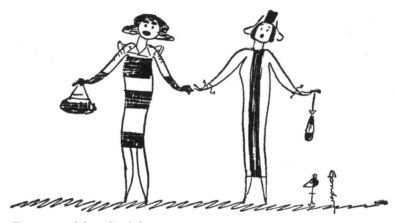

Every up-and-down line helps

cowl neckline is good, especially if you are tall. And, speaking of necklines, be careful of any necklace you may wear. Avoid chokers or any necklace that merely encircles the neck. They will only make you look heavier. Your necklaces should be longer.

Now descend to your waistline. First, be careful of belts. In general, it is well to have them match or blend into your frock. Contrasting belts, especially wide or bright ones, will merely emphasize the width you want to hide. Never wear a contrasting buckle or a tied belt that fastens in a little bow. Leave those X-marks-the-spot details to slender gals. Your belts should be worn to fit your waist, neither tight nor loose.

Your sleeves should be fairly straight, generously cut at the shoulders, and not too short. In fact, unless your arms are thin in proportion to the rest of you, short sleeves should be avoided. If you have pretty hands, rings will be becoming; but if your hands are fat, it would be just as well not to call attention to them by wearing attractive rings.

The mode for extra jackets on sports things, day ensembles, and evening clothes is excellent for you. A straight jacket of about fingertip length will do much for your figure. But do not have it in a contrasting color. Let it match the frock with which you wear it.

Your coats should be unbelted and should not have fluffy fur collars, unless you are that tall, fine figure of a woman.

What colors should you wear? Black, of course, is always perfect. So, too, are "grayed" colors—slate blues, dusty pastels, grayed greens. If you wear a fabric with a print in it, be sure it is a small symmetrical print, a small check, or lengthwise stripes. Splashy prints and crosswise stripes are bad. And always wear dull fabrics. No matter how much you may like satin, don't yield to that temptation. Nothing makes one look stouter than a fabric which catches all the highlights. Very stiff fabrics are bad, too. A soft, fairly heavy crêpe; a very heavy triple-sheer; a thin wool; are safest and always smart. If you combine two fabrics in one dress, be very careful. On the whole, it is safer to stick to one fabric and one color. For eveningwear, lace is excellent. It is soft, flattering, and almost universally becoming. When it is in the mode, by all means use it for your more formal clothes.

If your face is large, keep away from tiny hats. Choose medium-width brims, preferably with a slightly irregular line or with trimming or emphasis on one side. Evenly balanced hats tend to make the face look fuller.

Keep your hair well-groomed and not too fluffy. Never wear it cut very short. You must be careful of your grooming. See that your hands are well cared for, your heels always straight. And, by the way, do not wear terribly high heels unless you have particularly attractive ankles. Heavy legs look twice as heavy above a high, spike heel.

So often an easygoing disposition goes with a few extra pounds. You plump ladies tend to have an added measure of graciousness. Remember this when you consider dieting. If being on a diet makes you jumpy and irritable, it probably isn't worth your effort. Everyone prefers a few extra pounds to a shrewish disposition. But, if a little judicious dieting and a little exercise can take off some of your weight, you will doubtless be rewarded by those sweetest of all words, "How well you're looking—and so much younger, too."

Color can play tricks

In the somewhat general advice we have just given you, there was a brief mention of color. But color is a fashion factor that deserves closer study. No woman can look her best unless she is careful of her colors.

"But I have no color sense," or, "I never know what to combine with what." These are plaints we often hear. Nonsense! You don't need an artist's trained eye or a stylist's taste to find the things that look best on you.

When you think back to a particularly successful dress or hat, do you merely say, "That blue dress was a joy. Everyone told me how well I looked whenever I wore it"? Or do you remember that it was the narrow white collar that did the trick—and do you plan another dress with a similar touch of white? You should, of course. Profit by your successes by repeating them in a slightly different version. Profit by your mistakes by never making them a second time.

If you have color prejudices, examine them carefully before you allow them to control your buying. For instance, we know a girl who is somewhat mousy in coloring. She has nondescript brown hair, eyes neither blue nor gray, regular features that are not particularly striking in either a good or a bad way. Just a face, in other words. We were looking through some fabric swatches with her.

"This sheer gray wool would be grand on you."

"On me?" she asked incredulously. "I never wear gray. I'm too colorless myself."

"Not at all. Your skin is just tan enough in tone to be wonderful with gray." And we finally persuaded her to get a dress-length of the fabric.

Later, she appeared in the frock. Before we had a chance to get a good look at her, we knew the dress was a success. Her walk proclaimed the fact that she was wearing something that she *knew* was becoming. Compliments had already been raising their pretty heads.

"Hello, Jeanne—ah, the new gray dress—and *very* lovely, too. You never looked better in your life."

"I don't quite understand it," she murmured. "I never wore gray before."

"Well, you'll wear it again, you may be sure."

Never had that girl's skin looked so golden and smooth, never had her eyes looked so clear and gray. She had suddenly acquired color—by wearing gray! That's what we mean by a color trick.

Black magic

What color shall you wear? Before we discuss colors for various types, we must say a word about black. Almost every woman looks well in it. But "black" may mean many things. To the ultra-chic *Parisienne,* it means a dress of exquisite fabric, intricate cut, and simple effect. She wears it with costly jewels and a sophisticated hat. In it, she is her smartest and characteristic self.

But, unless you have the price of very expensive clothes, this isn't the sort of "black" we want to talk about. We mean the simple little black frock that is a lifesaver for dozens of occasions. You can wear it countless times. You will not tire of it as quickly as you will of that gay print or that wine crêpe. And your friends will not have the feeling of repetition if they see it dozens of times. That is, they won't, if you use your ingenuity a bit.

Here are a few things to do to a simple black frock to give it the spice of variety:

(1) If it is a dress with a collar, have two or three collars in different colors and alternate them. Be sure at least

one is white; for there is still nothing in the world more "appetizing" than a black dress with a fresh white collar.

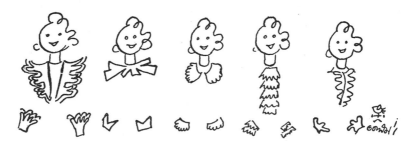

Have several collars . . .

(2) If it is a collarless dress, vary it with colorful scarfs. This doesn't mean rushing to a shop and buying a handful. Be a critical collector of scarfs. When Aunt Mary asks you what you want for your birthday, ask for a scarf. If you see an extraordinary bargain, treat yourself to it. If you make your own clothes, or have them made, remember that the leftover fabric of that pretty sheer or that attractive print will make a good little triangle to knot softly at the neck of your black frock. And remember that many women who think they can't wear black would find it enormously becoming if they would just wear a dash of color with it.

(3) If it is a frock with a very simple blouse, you can often wear a plastron or "topper" over it. These should be chosen with greatest care. If you are slender, white is always

effective. But if you are inclined to be somewhat chesty, choose a soft, dull color. If you are really large around the bust, do not use this particular way to camouflage your black frock.

(4) Jewelry is another means to variety. A necklace of several strands of pearls will make a black dress look more formal and dressy. A necklace of gold or silver (with or without colored stones) is less formal but equally attractive. Strings of colored beads (they can be very inexpensive; just be sure their color is becoming) will work wonders. Or use a pair of nice clips, instead of any of the necklaces.

(5) One of the best tricks is to add a gay little jacket to a black frock. If your print ensemble has a black background with bright flowers or a colored background with plenty of black in the pattern, by all means try the jacket over your black dress. If you cannot decide whether you like it, try hanging them together on a coat hanger and placing them where you can step away and examine them. If you saw them together in a shop, would you buy them? If so, by all means wear them together. If not, scout around for another jacket. It may be the bolero of your evening frock, or an extra jacket which you can buy or make yourself.

A word of warning about your black clothes. Don't forget that they need frequent cleaning. Because the dust and grime do not show so much, women sometimes think that their black frocks can be worn indefinitely without a trip to the cleaner. That's a bad blunder, and one which may eventually prove costly. It may cost you the esteem, or even the friendship, of a fastidious person who detects that musty unpleasant odor which clings to clothes that need cleaning.

What goes with what?

One problem which is often mentioned may be summarized in the plaint of Betty S. who said sadly, "I know I look best in navy blue, but I get so tired of it. If I could just be sure what colors to use with it, I'd be all right."

Betty, and all you countless others who look well in navy blue, here are the colors that look best with it: navy with white, soft pink, sharp green, lemon yellow, lighter blue, bright red, dull purple, wine red. Surely there's enough variety for anyone!

Let's consider the dark brown that so often gains vitality by having a bit of contrast—brown with soft green, a light dull blue, dusty pink, beige, copper, yellow, white. And, if you can trust your color sense, certain browns with certain grays.

With green—we're talking of the dark soft green that you would choose for a woolen frock—use contrast carefully. But you would be safe with brown, chartreuse, soft rust, soft yellow, bright red, black.

What goes best with gray? Yellow, white, darkish brown, black, bright red, dull green, navy, a touch of purple.

What colors shall you wear?

It is not easy to prescribe colors. Hair, skin tone, and eyes are the three important factors to consider. One cannot generalize and say, if you are a blonde wear so-and-so. A blonde with white skin and pale blue eyes may look obvious in yellow, while another with amber-toned skin and dark eyes looks enchanting in it.

But there is far too much hocus-pocus about this whole subject. Almost anyone can wear almost any color, if she will exercise a little common sense.

If you think you look sallow in green, put on a tiny bit of extra rouge. If you think brown makes you a little colorless, be generous with your lipstick. The way to find out is to experiment. And if you're not altogether sure, ask a friend whose color sense is acute.

In general, these are becoming colors for various types:

Every blonde looks well in black. Blue is good, and so is brown, beige, green, yellow (not too light or bright), white, dusty pink, and gray.

Brunettes with light skin look well in black. Brunettes with dark or sallow skin may need a touch of color with their black. They usually find becoming colors among the sharp blues, the greens, reds, and brown. They can wear white, of course, yellow, beige, and a soft raisin shade.

Redheads know that they look well in greens and browns. But let them adventure a bit into the fields of gray, beige, white, yellow, navy, and black.

Gray-haired women look most charming in black, white, soft blue, brown, navy, gray (with either black or white), and black with a dash of emerald green.

If you are very fond of a color, but you find that it does nothing for you, satisfy your liking for it by using it in small doses, in combination with a color that you know is becoming. And one last word, unless you feel happy in a color, leave it for others. Never wear a color merely because it is smart.

Do you plan or do you plunge?

If you could see Mrs. M. and Mrs. B., you would have living models of the right and wrong way to shop for clothes.

Mrs. M. is wealthy, she spends a great deal on her clothes, she buys only the best. Is she chic? She is not. She misses it by a mile! Last winter, on Fifth Avenue, she was seen wearing a regal mink coat over a reddish brown dress that was just the wrong shade; a hat with too wide a brim, that interfered with the line of her coat collar; beige gloves that were too pink in tone. Yet each individual item was, by itself, costly and correct.

Mrs. B., whom we chanced to meet a few days later, was wearing a well-fitted black cloth coat, with a sleek little black turban, chamois gloves, and soft yellow and gray scarf, knotted loosely and tucked into the neck of her collarless coat. She looked as though she had stepped from the show-window of a smart shop. Yet her income is small and she also has to dress two children on her very limited budget.

What is the answer? Planning, of course—careful, thoughtful planning.

Planning a wardrobe

How does one go about it? Many women's magazines have a blissful way of attacking the problem as though money grew on trees. They tell you how many dresses and pairs of shoes you will need, what hats and coats to choose, and what accessories. But most of us cannot afford a whole new wardrobe at one time. And even women who could afford it would think twice before they threw out a few favorite frocks or a good coat and started from scratch.

Planning begins at home, right in front of your clothes closet. But even before that, there is one important step. Sit down for a moment and think. During the coming season, where will you be going, what will you be doing? Exactly what type of clothes will you need the most?

If you are a businesswoman, you should give extra care to your office clothes.

If you are a housewife whose chief dissipation is bridge, have a few very pretty afternoon frocks.

If you are a woman who goes in for club activities, be sure you have at least two good daytime dresses and the right hats to wear with them.

If you go to many dances with the same crowd of friends, be as thrifty as possible on your day clothes and have delectable evening frocks.

If you spend a great deal of time on your feet, have the best and most comfortable shoes, even though you may have to economize elsewhere.

No one except you can plan your wardrobe. But here are a few general ideas which may help:

Let's get back to your clothes closet. Take out everything you have left from last year. Let us suppose that it is an autumn and winter wardrobe you are planning. Out comes the old coat (how bored you are with it!), the crêpe frock, the brown wool street dress, the tired dinner gown, the suit that was such a bargain but really not much fun to wear. What a collection! This is the time when familiarity breeds contempt. You'd like to bundle them all up and send them to a worthy charity. But you can't. So sit down and do the next best thing.

If you can sew, you're in luck. If you've never tried to sew, by all means make an effort. Or, if you don't want to sew, find an inexpensive seamstress. You have no idea how much money you can save if you've never tried this most practical of all ways to use leftovers.

Well, that old coat. You really do need a new one. But let's not make a decision about it until we've considered the whole problem. Put the coat aside for a moment. If you can manage to salvage the suit, perhaps you'll be able to get that much-needed coat. Your suit wasn't a success. The skirt was never becoming because it bulged in back, though you did like the jacket. And it was a good-looking tweed. How about the old wool dress? You never realized how nice its plain brown surface looks next to that nubby green tweed. Why not make a new skirt out of the wool dress? Sometimes that merely means cutting at the waistline and mounting the skirt on a belt. Sometimes it means a complete remaking. But even that is less expensive than buying a new skirt.

Well, if that works, you won't have to spend much on a suit. So there's something saved toward that new coat.

How about the crêpe dress? Is it beyond redemption? Well, it's black and that's a help. But the collar looks worn and gray. Cleaning can't change that. How about ripping off the collar entirely and putting on a small one of heavy white silk? Don't sew it in. Put it on with snaps, so that you can remove it easily. Why not have several collars? A dusty pink or a soft yellow would be lovely on black, if those colors look well on you. At any rate, the old black crêpe will do to *start* the season. So again you've saved something toward the coat.

The dinner gown is a lovely color, but you've worn it so often. And its skirt has a decidedly last-year look. Must you wear it another season? No—you have a plan. You'll get a coat. It will be black, because your last one was brown and also because the wardrobe that includes only one coat can stretch itself furthest on black. You'll ask the store to get you enough extra fabric from the manufacturer to make a simple skirt. The neighborhood tailor will make it for you for very little. The old dinner gown can then be cut up to make a really lovely blouse to wear with the new skirt. And you doubtless have other blouses or sweaters that will do nicely with the black skirt and give you a well-put-together look when you wear them with the new black coat.

That leaves a dinner gown to be bought. And, when you get some extra money, a street dress or two. That is the way to plan.

Of course, your closet will doubtless reveal an entirely different set of props, but the theory holds just the same. Too many women look dowdy merely because they do not make the effort to pull their wardrobes into shape. It does take thought and effort. But the results more than justify them. Chic can easily be a triumph of mind over money.

Buyer beware!

Are you a bargain buyer? Then beware. This way danger lies. Of course, occasionally one can find a bargain that is just perfect. It fits into your general plan and it fits you. Its price is reasonable, so grab it.

But, no matter how beguiling the price tag, think before you say "I'll take it." Relate the object, mentally, to the things you already have.

If it's a dress, consider the coat and hat you'll be wearing with it. How about your shoes and purse? If there's no harmony ahead, your pet bargain will soon become your prize eyesore. Be strong. Drop it, as though it had thorns. Watch for another bargain that will really be worth its purchase price.

If it's a hat, be sure that it will live in sympathy with the clothes you have, and with your face. While it is undeniable that a giddy, extreme hat may work wonders on the morale, its effect is temporary. If you can afford such a luxury, by all means have it. But if you have to wear and wear your things, it's better to lean toward the more conservative bonnets. That does not necessarily mean the conventional little felt with nothing but safety to offer. It merely means avoiding the too-bizarre, the too-dashing styles. When high crowns are smart, by all means have one. It needn't tower to dizzy faddish heights. Leave extremes to the ladies who do not have to live with their mistakes.

What is simplicity?

There's no point in shrugging your shoulders and saying, "Everybody knows what simplicity is." Look around you. How many people are dressed with any degree of simplicity? Too much trimming on the dress, too much gingerbread on the shoes, too much jewelry, too many artificial flowers—these are prevalent maladies.

One of the most important definitions of simplicity is "restraint." Not severity, but restraint. If the dress is absolutely plain in cut, it can take a colorful necklace or a bright scarf. If it has a complicated neckline, don't add more complications by wearing a necklace. Perhaps this dress needs merely a good-looking bracelet or earrings.

Before you leave your own room, it's always well to take a quick look in the mirror. Is there an extra something you can take off? Some bit of trimming or a one-too-many piece of jewelry?

You can't hurt your costume by eliminating trimming
details. Be ruthless and you will be simple. Be simple and
you'll go a long way toward chic.

Accessories speak volumes

Accessories are a giveaway. They tell volumes about you,
your taste, your judgment.

Go to your bureau or dressing table and take out
every purse and belt, every scarf and pair of gloves. Go
to your closet and take out every hat and every pair of
shoes. Look them over. Are they accessories that lift
an ordinary costume into the realm of smartness, or
are they detractors and hangers-on that do more harm
than good?

Don't buy your accessories helter-skelter. "That's a
sweet purse" . . . "this belt's a bargain" . . . "pretty gloves,
aren't they?" That's not the way to decide!

When you add up the cost of all the extras that go to
make up even a simple costume, you may be staggered by
the total. That's why each part should be selected with
an eye to its fitness not only for this one ensemble, but
for many others, too.

There are two schools of thought about accessories.
One school believes that only the best will do. The second
maintains that the trick is to have a lot of inexpensive

accessories to give you plenty of variety. We disagree with both schools.

Here's our plan: Have two or three complete sets of accessories, as costly as you can afford without overtaxing your budget. Have them of sufficiently good quality so that they will stand up under frequent use. Buy them as carefully as you would your best evening gown.

Permit yourself an occasional frippery, if you wish. An inexpensive, colorful cotton purse for summer use, a gay belt that will look well with one or two frocks only (and will therefore not be worn with any others), a giddy pair of earrings or clips that turn your simple black dress into a thing to be noticed. These occasional sprees are good, of course. But it's like dieting. When you break your diet, let it be for a very special treat. It's the consistent little lapses that add the pounds! And in buying, it's those lapses that rob you of money for the smart necessities.

Recently a magazine devoted a page to the idea . . . "Give your black frock variety." It showed the black dress in the center of the page and then showed, in the four corners, four complete sets of accessories—shoes, purses, belts, gloves, even handkerchiefs. We feel that is a trick, neither realistic nor helpful, and a far cry from the variety we mentioned before. Any woman who can afford four pairs of shoes and four purses for one dress can afford more than one dress!

Far cleverer is the woman who buys an excellent navy blue purse and belt for her spring suit, and then plans a midsummer ensemble of a linen or heavy cotton in white, or natural, or pink—any of which would look well with navy accessories. By stretching their use, she gives herself more to spend for clothes.

No one can tell you just which things to buy or how much to pay for them. But if you will think before you buy, and if you will relate each item to the various clothes with which you will be wearing it, you will avoid costly mistakes in choosing these "tremendous trifles."

There's danger in their lines

Do you remember the popular song, "There's Danger in Your Eyes, Chérie"? Try to remember it and paraphrase it—especially at the moment when the saleswoman stands behind you with her hands upraised and chants, "That hat looks lovely on you." Take a hand mirror and look at the hat and at your face and hair, from both sides, and from the back. Stand up and walk toward the mirror. Try to see yourself, and your hat-to-be, as others will see you.

If you feel like a fool in it, don't take it, even though it's smart as can be. On the other hand, don't be afraid to try hats that are different from the kind you usually wear. It is hard to tell which is worse in buying a hat—the too-daring mood or the too-conservative. You must try to be brave, but not foolhardy.

If you are a woman who has her hair done regularly, who wears it in the newest, smartest fashion and keeps it always perfectly groomed, then you can afford to be a bit dashing and original in your choice. For, even if the hat is not the most flattering in the world, it may well give you an air of sophisticated chic that can be better than mere prettiness. But if you are casual about your coiffure and have it done only on occasion, try to choose hats that look "at home" and flattering when your hair is in its average state.

One woman we know has an unfailing sense about choosing her headgear. We asked her for her rules. Here they are:

1. I buy one good hat every season—the best I can afford. Then I fill in with an occasional inexpensive hat or one that I pick up in a sale. But I always have one dependable standby.

2. I always buy hats on days when I look my worst. Then I'm pleasantly surprised when I wear them. If you buy a hat when you're looking your best and have just had your hair set, you're due for disappointment when you give it run-of-the-mill wearing.

3. I never buy a hat in a hurry. It's one thing that needs studying from all angles. Impulsive hat purchases are too often disastrous.

And there you are. Simple as that!

Well-groomed, we say

"She always looks charming—so well-groomed." That's one side of the picture. The reverse is, "Why doesn't Jane ever look smart?—she spends plenty on her clothes."

Nine chances out of ten, the difference is a mere matter of grooming. Grooming, of course, includes everything from well-kept fingernails to straight heels. But let us consider, for the moment, only matters of dress.

Suppose you buy your clothes readymade. Before you wear them, you should inspect every detail carefully to see that:

1. All snaps and buttons are firmly sewed.
2. All loose threads are cut off. (Knot them first, so that seams will not open.)
3. All plackets are flat and firmly closed. Often you will need to sew a few extra snaps or hooks and eyes *between* the ones that are there, to avoid that unpleasant spectacle—a grinning placket. Slide fasteners do away with this, too.

4. If there is a belt, it fits you snugly. A loose belt will
sag and spoil even the best of figures.

5. If cuffs are too loose or sleeves too baggy, they are
altered. A badly fitted sleeve will ruin any dress.

6. The hem is even and your skirt does not sag in
the back.

These six precautions may take a little time, but once
they're taken, they're taken for good. And you can't be well-
groomed unless you watch these things.

What men think about grooming

We asked several well-known men about town what they
considered the worst offense against good grooming.

Their list included everything from wavy seams in
stockings to fussing with your back curls. But three points
seemed sufficiently universal to warrant special mention.
They are:

1. *The runaway shoulder straps.* You've probably gone digging for them countless times; we all have. The strap of
your slip or bra slides off your shoulder and you try to
retrieve it with that unmistakable groping gesture. Avoid
this. The remedy is so simple. Sew lingerie loops into the
shoulders of every dress you wear. These little loops come
on cards and may be purchased in the chain stores. They
take only a moment to sew in. Then, when you dress, you

slip your shoulder straps under the loop and snap it. The straps are then firmly anchored until you release them. A little thing, but what a difference it can make!

2. *The peeping slip.* "Your slip is showing."

"Oh dear! I *did* knot those shoulder straps this morning—they must have opened again."

Yes, that's the story we've all told at one time or another. But hitching up the shoulder straps isn't the answer. If the slip is too long, shorten it. Shorten it from the bottom. See that it hangs evenly all around, and stays invisible under your shortest frock. Move around a bit when you're deciding how much to take off, because action sometimes changes the hang of your skirt. You can't look charming with dangling underwear, so watch your slip!

3. *The overstuffed purse.* "I have everything but the kitchen stove in here," laughs a lady as she digs into her overcrowded handbag. Judging from the comments of several gentlemen, I know they have no liking for this particular feminine weakness. Here are a few of their words of wisdom:

"When I see a purse that's bulging with junk, I always think of an untidy person and a poor housekeeper."

"No matter how neat a woman looks, a sloppy, overfilled handbag is a dead giveaway. I know her bureau drawers are a mess. And I suspect her mind is, too."

"I hate to see a woman hunting in a full purse for a handkerchief and then retrieve it with little flecks of tobacco clinging to it."

Perhaps these remarks will make you give your handbags regular inspection. Tear up those odd scraps of paper, throw away the rumpled piece of Kleenex, brush out the tobacco crumbs and the traces of powder, clean your comb, wipe the red rim off your lipstick. There! Now your purse is ready to be seen in public. And, what's more, you'll find your things without digging.

Heads up!

But, aside from all these details, what do we mean when we say "well-groomed?" A woman who looks fresh and clean, who smells nice, who wears becoming clothes that go together harmoniously, a woman who spends considerable time and thought on putting herself together—and then forgets about it when she's finished.

It is the forgetting that contributes so greatly to real poise. The woman who wonders whether she's coming apart in the middle or whether there's a hole in the heel of her stocking, is usually so engrossed in these petty details that she can't be at ease in any social relationship. That's why it is so important to do your grooming thoroughly and competently. Only then does it recede into its proper place in the background.

The greatest pianist cannot make beautiful music on a piano that is out of tune. You cannot relax and be at your best when there is some trivial but disturbing detail to distract you.

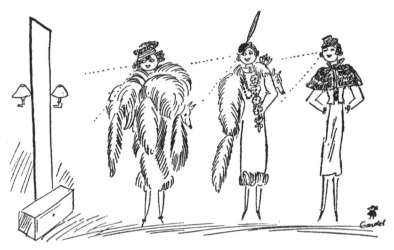

Look before you leave

So, stand in front of your mirror. Look before you leave. Get yourself pulled together, and then sally forth armed with self-confidence and assurance.

That is the secret of poise—the poise that makes you hold your head erect—the poise that makes people notice you, listen to you, admire you.

Part Two:

WHAT YOU DO TO
OTHERS

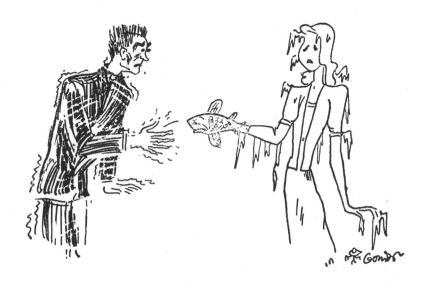

4   *First Impressions*

HAVE a heart of gold, by all means, but don't expect it to help you very much when you first meet people. Forget all the old maxims about not judging a book by its cover, and remember that first impressions *must* be surface impressions. And when you save the surface, you may be well on the way to saving all! So, put your very best self forward and make the first impression a favorable one. Later on, let your intelligence and your integrity get in their good work.

Shaking hands

Do you like to touch a dead fish? Who does? When you offer your hand in greeting, be sure it carries a warm, firm grip, not a slithery, flabby, come-and-get-me droop. Shake hands as though you were genuinely pleased to meet the person.

When should you shake hands? Whenever that seems a natural and easy gesture. Etiquette books may lay down rigid rules, but the safest one to follow is— be natural. If you are introduced to a man in a business office, it is not necessary to shake hands. If you are in a restaurant, you would not reach across the table to shake hands. If you are being introduced at a large party, it is simpler merely to nod and smile and say "How do you do?" than it is to get from one person to another. But if a friend of yours is presenting a friend of his, it is perfectly correct to extend your hand in a cordial greeting.

Never be afraid of doing the wrong thing. Whatever is courteous and pleasant is bound to be right. And, once and forever, discard the notion that people are watching you to see whether or not you are being correct. Do you watch others and pick flaws in their behavior? Of course you don't. Who cares?

You can forget the Do's and Don'ts of etiquette, if you will set up this simple standard . . . *the only bad manners are those which are unkind or which contribute to another person's discomfort.*

There are smiles . . .

Just as important as the gesture of shaking hands is the facial expression that accompanies it. You have often seen people with an artificial grin—one that looks as though you could wipe it off with a wave of the hand. How you dislike it! A smile must have warmth as well as width. Haven't you often seen poor skin and irregular features completely counteracted by an attractive smile?

And, while we're talking of smiles, think a moment about the way people laugh. Raucous shouts, silly giggles, forced and affected laughter—how unpleasant these can be. And how we all respond to a hearty, genuine laugh. It doubles the enjoyment of a joke. It creates a gratifying bond between people; it can cement a relationship faster than many words.

So don't be afraid to laugh. Everyone likes people who enjoy things and who are not afraid to show their enjoyment. There's nothing quite as paralyzing and chilling as the woman who wears an expression which says "I dare you to amuse me." People soon give up the task and seek more responsive fields.

Your tone of voice

Many a woman is attractive until she talks. Then a shrill voice or a nasal twang or a deadly drawl may completely spoil the picture.

Can you hear yourself talk? Yes, you can, if you will take the trouble. Talk out loud when you're alone. Anyone who stumbles in upon this performance will wonder what has happened to you, but never mind that. Is your voice harsh? Then talk in an exaggeratedly soft tone. Is it shrill? Then pitch it so low that it seems to come out of your shoes.

If you find that you can't hear your own voice, the next best thing is to corner one of your good friends. Choose someone whose taste and judgment you respect, someone who is sufficiently fond of you to be honest and to be willing to work with you. Ask if your voice is pleasant. Ask her to tell you exactly what it needs to make it so. And then practice. Practice with her, and when you are alone.

Your voice is worth working with. People are repelled, sometimes consciously, sometimes unconsciously, by an unpleasant voice. And who can estimate the aura of charm which is induced by a well-modulated voice?

What is an "outgoing person"?

"I like Anne—she's so outgoing." You've heard that kind of comment many a time. But have you ever stopped to think about what an outgoing person is? One who is interested in other people and in the things which happen to them? Yes—but this does not mean a person who gossips about other people's affairs, not one who gushes over everyone. It means an interest which is all wool and a yard wide.

Some people ask "How are you?" and, while you tell them, their minds are wandering to something else, or they are thinking of the next bright remark they plan to make. Do not ask how people are unless you want to know and intend to give them the courtesy of your undivided attention while they answer your question.

People often talk to you about things which interest them, but do not interest you. Their children, their stamp collection, their garden—these may be of vital importance to them. So give them an audience until you've heard the whole story and can then painlessly switch to another subject of more general interest. It is unforgivable to break in with an anecdote which concerns *your* pet hobby or *your* children. And don't think that you can let your thoughts wander, without having your victims feel it. Better a few moments of boredom than an exhibition of discourtesy. We all like to have an audience when we talk, so let's not be too prone to think that the other fellow's tale is dull and our own is dazzling.

But, far deeper than a mere matter of listening, is the interest in others which marks the truly outgoing person. When you feel very much put upon because something goes wrong with your scheme of things, remember that everyone has hardships and annoyances. One look at mass problems of unemployment, hunger, drought, and persecution will give you a gauge by which to measure your own tribulations. Nine chances out of ten, your problems will take their proper place and you will see how relatively unimportant they are. Keep an open mind and an open eye on what is happening in the world; that's a sure way to be "outgoing."

Your troubles are yours

But, granted that you have troubles, genuine ones, what place should they assume in your scheme of social relationships?

How do you like the woman who greets you with, "Oh, the most dreadful thing happened to me the other day . . ."

Or the one who, when you say, "How well you're looking," answers with, "Well, I may *look* well, but I really don't feel a bit well . . . my back has been bothering me terribly . . ." Or the one who pants, "There's something I simply *must* tell you about Jerry . . ." Then you know you're in for a session of hearing about her love life.

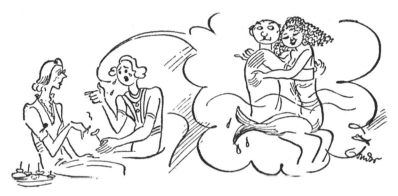

"I simply must *tell you about Jerry . . ."*

It is always unwise to tell your troubles—physical, mental, or spiritual—to a casual acquaintance. You have no right to assume any interest on the other person's part. Those are your problems, not hers, and it is your job to solve them.

That doesn't mean that you should not enlist the sympathetic interest of a friend. That's what friends are for. But before you spill it even to a close friend, be sure that she can be truly helpful. If your problems are economic, you can expect no practical advice from a friend whose income is fabulous. If you are disturbed by some husband-wife difficulty, don't talk to the friend who has had two divorces, and tells you that repair work is impossible.

In other words, choose your confidante with care. Will she be able to evaluate the whole situation? Will she be open-minded? Has she the wisdom in human relationships to be able to deal frankly with you and tell you a few unpleasant truths, if that is what you need? If she has these qualities, tell her all the details as you would describe your physical symptoms to a doctor, and then discuss your problem from every angle. But if she is the sort of person who habitually makes mountains out of molehills, avoid her as you would the plague. You can do your own magnifying without any assistance. What you want is a balanced, sane point of view, with plenty of perspective.

Omit the terrible details

Even more boring than the person who tells her troubles is the person who smothers every anecdote under a mountain of irrelevant details.

When you tell a story, remember that brevity always was and always will be the soul of wit. Cut away all the unimportant trivia that can strangle even the brightest story. Some women tell a story in this manner: "The other day,

I saw the most amusing thing in the bus. I was riding down-town on Wednesday—no it was Thursday—no, that's right, it *was* Wednesday—in the Madison Avenue bus—no, it was Lexington because I remember passing Bloomingdales' and thinking how attractive their windows looked . . . well, a man got on . . ." But by this time your interest in the anec-dote is nonexistent. It made no difference what day of the week it was, nor which bus line. The point of the story did not require this elaborate preparation. When you tell a story, or express an opinion, try to say only those things which contribute to the matter at hand. *Cut it short!*

And please don't be a tangent talker—the woman who starts telling a story and, halfway through, changes to another topic. Here's a fair sample of her conversation: "Did you hear that new radio program last night—the one about the two women . . . sort of reminded me of the time Jack and I decided to take Donnie to see the . . . . Oh! by the way, Donnie brought home his report card yesterday—it really showed quite an improvement. His teacher—she's a cute little blonde—her brother is an air pilot . . ."

Hopelessly trailing behind, you're still wondering what the radio program was about and what Donnie's teacher's brother has to do with the case.

Exaggerated? No. Listen carefully to some of the casual chatter you hear at home, or at a friend's house, or on a bus.

People's tales wander because their thinking wanders. Straight talking is the result of straight thinking.

Before you can talk

Before you can talk, you must have something to talk about. Does this seem too obvious to need statement? Not when you hear the aimless chatter that floats around. What do these people read, what do they think about? Do they think? Are they aware that this is a fast-changing world?

It is difficult to give a recipe for successful conversation. But it would certainly include three fundamentals. Assemble good ingredients, mix and spice with your own thinking, and serve attractively.

To assemble the ingredients, read. Read lots of different things. Read newspapers that express a viewpoint contrary to your own; read periodicals that have thoughtful, provocative articles; read books that tell of places and persons of current interest; read fiction, of course, but not to the exclusion of all other things.

If you do not have time to read your newspapers thoroughly, at least read all the headlines and subheads carefully. They give you the news in capsule form. Then read as many of the articles as you have time or inclination for.

If you miss part of the week's news, try to see the résumé in the newspapers at the end of the week; or one of the newsmagazines.

But, of course, mere facts are insufficient ingredients unless they are seasoned by opinions and mixed with imagination. Nothing is duller than the talk of a walking encyclopedia.

You have met the woman who tells you that it takes exactly fifteen and three-quarters hours to get from Newark to Los Angeles in one of the new planes. She

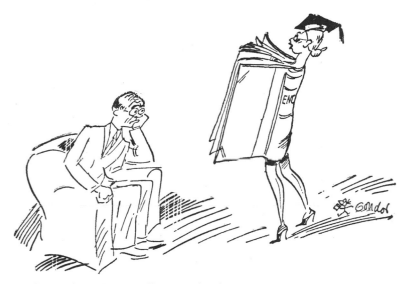

Nothing is duller than a walking encyclopedia

reminds you of the difference in time, too—and right to the minute. But you feel sure that it makes little difference whether she be on the East Coast or the West. She'll miss the fun while she coddles the facts. And you know the man who tells you that the stars are so-and-so many million light-miles away. You'd never choose him for a stroll in a moonlit garden—not a second time, anyway.

Occasionally we do meet that rare soul who has a line of small talk that is diverting and amusing. But those people are few and far between. Most of us need to replenish our stock with the information we glean elsewhere.

The most interesting talk usually contains a lively exchange of opinions. Not dogmatic statements delivered in the tone of an oracle, but opinions. A willingness to express what you think and then consider the opposing point of view. A willingness to listen quietly and talk quietly. Shouting an opinion doesn't make it more emphatic. On the contrary, try to remember the man who said, with truth, "Don't talk so loudly, I can't hear you." Your audience automatically shuts its ears against the noise and its mind against the opinion.

And it is a good thing to know where you stand on the important issues of the day. Do not have the idea that you need to be a statesman or a lawyer to know whether a certain trend is vicious or helpful. After all, there is no great mystery about most things. Use common sense when you judge an issue. Is it something which will be advantageous to a few and harmful to many? If it is, do you need legal training to reject it? Try to read the news with an eye for possible propaganda. Try to see what's *behind* the articles you read.

One of the most boring and unsatisfactory of conversationalists is the person who shies away from any serious discussion. If you mention an important struggle between

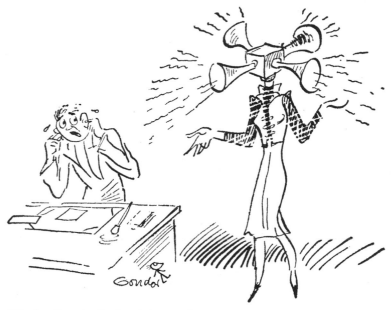

"Don't talk so loudly, I can't hear you"

two factions (whether they be political groups, or capital and labor), she will shrug her shoulders and, "Oh, I don't know anything about it. I think it would be a good idea

to put them all in a big arena and let them fight it out."
How revealing such a statement is! In the first place, she
should know something about it. In the second place, she
should care who wins, because there is nothing in the world
which, sooner or later, will not affect every human being.
Know what's happening. And know where you stand.

What you talk about

What should you talk about? The things that interest your
listeners as well as yourself. If you have a hobby, talk of it,
by all means. But as soon as you see attention wandering,
drop it and turn to other topics.

The woman who loves her garden, for example, can
talk to you gayly about the experiences she has with it. She
can be interesting, even though you may not care about
gardening yourself. But if she burdens you with technical
talk which could only appeal to a fellow horticulturist, she
is a bore.

If you know that your listener has a hobby, let him or
her bring it out and show it off. Even though you may not
care for the same thing, there may be some part of the subject which interests you or which furnishes a starting point
for other discussions or ideas.

In general, a good rule is don't talk about your health,
don't list your symptoms, don't tell in detail what you had
for lunch or breakfast or dinner at Elsie's last Wednesday.

"Elsie had a wonderful dinner when we were there. First we had tomato juice. Of course we really started with cocktails in the living room, with tiny rolled sandwiches of cheese and watercress. And then the tomato juice and we had steak and French fried potatoes and the green peas were those very tiny ones . . ." By now your listener will either be dead of starvation or certain that he will never eat again, depending on the length of time since his last meal. And you will have established a firm reputation for dull conversation.

And there's the breakfast-boaster. She belongs in one of two groups. Group one functions like this: "I never eat anything for breakfast except orange juice, toast, and coffee. And I just take one thin slice of toast with very little butter and no cream in my coffee." Group two usually regales you with, "I do enjoy my breakfast. It's the one meal of the day I *really* enjoy. I always have some sort of fruit, half a grapefruit or a dish of berries or something; then I have cereal, sometimes hot, sometimes cold; and a couple of eggs; and coffee and rolls—usually two rolls. Then I'm ready to start my day." And you're ready to call it a day and be done with it.

What is a good listener?

Strange as it may seem, a good listener isn't a person who sits and listens. That isn't enough. You must show by your face, your questions, your comments, that you're not merely listening with your ears, but with your mind. You must contribute to the conversation. If you cannot add ideas, you can do your part by having a genuinely wide-awake attitude which is active, not passive.

And do not interrupt. If someone is telling a joke or an anecdote to a group of people and you have already heard it, do not cut in with "Oh! I know that one." It takes the wind out of the storyteller's sails. But, on the contrary, if someone tells a story directly to you and you have heard it, by all means stop the person as soon as you recognize the tale. It's ever so much kinder than waiting to the end and then awarding it a feeble laugh.

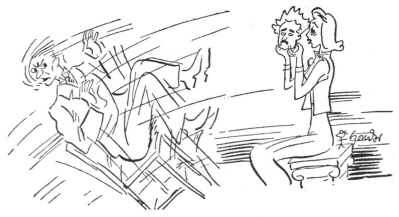

It isn't your Intelligence Quotient

5   *It's Not Your I.Q.*

IT'S one thing to make a good impression. It's another to bulwark that impression with a lasting reputation for charm. We can't go through life meeting, impressing, and parting. We meet people and then live much of our lives with them afterward. The scintillating personality that dazzles us all at a first meeting may or may not be considered fascinating after a third meeting. The beautiful newcomer may be a nine days' wonder and a great bore beyond that time. The famous writer or the less famous after-dinner speaker has a great advantage over the rest of us. One can make his bow without being present. The other needn't linger after he has impressed us with his wit.

But for the rest of us, first impressions are only first steps. We must build on the firm basis of relationships that wear well. We must have people like us, enjoy us day after day, feel comfortable with us, feel important and satisfied after being with us.

How do we do it? That is the real heart of the matter. All the externals of appearance merely smooth the way so that we can get in our durable work. It isn't a matter of brilliance, of greater education. It isn't your Intelligence Quotient. When people talk about Einstein's personality, it is often in a tone of wonder that one so brilliant should be so simple and so friendly.

"How on earth a woman can be as bright as she is, and still be such a fool, I don't know!" You've said it. You've heard others say it about some benighted female who has a talent for arrogance, or a genius for saying the worst thing at the worst time. She isn't just one of those lovable dimwits whose kind hearts usually compensate for their uncrowded heads. No, this woman is frequently a better-than-average thinker. Her career started in early grade school, where her marks were high and her popularity score was nil. And years of watching her "inferiors" walk off with the enviable jobs or invitations have not increased her affability.

We don't presume to say whether this woman can be changed. But she can be put under our microscope to determine what has made her someone to be tolerated but seldom sought after. It isn't brains this woman lacks. Usually, it is plain old-fashioned human kindness and an active imagination. She never knows that honest opinion is neither necessary nor kind. "I feel you ought to know . . ." is often the cruelest phrase in the language. It inevitably introduces the one piece of information that the recipient should *not* know. This woman has a passion for unpleasant truth that would give a psychiatrist something to work on.

To sum it up, she has no talent for human relations. A brutal self-analysis would reveal to her what *she* likes to be told, how *she* likes to have others see her, and would give her a quick guideline to what she should say and be to others.

How about you? Do you think people should be tough? That the toughening process is your job? Do you think people should understand what *you* mean, though you make no effort to understand how *they* feel? Do you discount the "empty headed" woman who nonetheless seems to attract the very people you hoped to interest? Then this is your chapter. And it also belongs to the overtimid woman who knows her I.Q. isn't too high, and worries over the social competition.

Consider young Betty B. By the intelligence test standards she was the dullest of "book learners." Betty couldn't retain a date more than a day. She had no business being in college. Yet she was captain of one team, manager of another, and one of the few winners of an award for the "best all-around girl." Fantastic? Perhaps. Still there wasn't a girl or boy on that campus who begrudged Betty the all-night sessions that pulled her through her exams, the written memos to keep her posted on game dates and places. Betty's presence at school was an addition. Her academic contribution was nonexistent. But there were brains enough to go around on that campus. The scarce qualities were consideration, loyalty, sweetness, sympathy. She had the kind of brains that could remember to mend a roommate's slip. She could dance gaily with the poorest dancer in the school, and never make a grimace at the stagline. She could think of just the right words to say to a self-conscious girl to make that girl bloom. Betty is no longer Miss B. She is a wife and mother known throughout a large circle for her gracious home, her lovely children, her tremendous charm.

Her talent isn't a vague thing. It can be rather easily charted. It is applied kindness. And it can be learned.

A simple thank-you

There is scarcely an hour that passes in which someone doesn't do something for you. It may be the grocery boy. It may be the mailman. Most of all, it will be the people with whom you work and live. Do you stop to realize the humanity of these givers of good things that make your life comfortable? Your telephone operator, your stenographer, your maid, your laundress, the man who tends your garden, the chauffeur who taxis you? What is your attitude toward them? Are they mere scenery, something you paid for and so needn't be aware of? You can't afford to think so. Your attitude toward those who serve you reflects your attitude toward everyone else. Charm springs from warmth, not etiquette.

"Thank-you" is a tribute, a recognition that we live by mutual aid and mutual consideration. Once you get this fundamental feeling that each of us lives by the grace of God and our fellowman, you will detect a new note in your thank-you. It ceases to be just a phrase. You stop wondering whether it is necessary to say it. It turns into graciousness and reflects itself in your every human contact.

Does this mean that you must be the wordy woman who embarrasses people by undue and false gratitude?

No, nor the over-enthusiastic bore who heaps grateful words upon the receipt of the most casual invitation. You have met her. She's the woman who accepts your hurried bridge suggestion with "Oh, my dear, how *nice* it is of you to think of us. We'd *love* to. And I know you have so many obligations. You're such a dear to think of me." Call her the poor-little-me type and dismiss her. She isn't gracious.

Neither do you want to join the ranks of the self-depreciators who reply to your compliment on a new hat, "Really do you like it? Of course I know a new hat is nothing to you, but I do so respect your judgment," etc., etc., ad infinitum. That woman is a public peril.

And so we emphasize the *simple* thank-you, free from elaboration, deprecation, abasement. The important thing is your own awareness of those who have helped you, in however small a measure. All the gratitude and gracious-ness that any normal occasion evokes can be dealt with by those two words. But never let them become routine. And never forget them.

The pseudojudiciary

Men call us cats, and do us an injustice. But if we dislike the description, why don't we get rid of the conversational habits that make us *seem* disloyal? Women have a meaning-less habit of assuming the judicial attitude. We label it "pseudojudicial" because it gives the victim no chance to

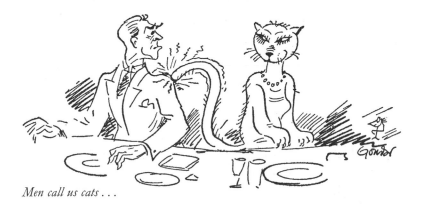

Men call us cats . . .

take the stand in her own defense. Women are prone to this cruel sport. We get a false sense of intimacy with our immediate companion when we sit in judgment upon an absent friend. It is so easy to be superior to the foibles that beset the absent member, as we tear her to pieces with the softest of words. It is easy to be sophisticated and witty, as we suggest grave or minor trespasses on her part.

We usually start out with a compliment to show how fair we are. "Maud is certainly a competent woman." "Yes, she always makes me feel shallow because she is 'above' clothes." "I don't see why you should feel that way. Maud could be just as capable and still pay a little more attention to her clothes." "Did you *see* that hat she had on the other day?" And so it goes. It winds up usually with a foreboding note that Maud "had better watch out or some little blonde will walk away with her husband." A man listening in would

have a right to assume that both women thoroughly dislike
Maud. A Freudian would insist that the women were
jealous of Maud who has a nice husband. And neither
would be right. The women like Maud. They don't feel
very strongly about her clothes or her competence or her
husband. They don't dream for a moment that a blonde
will break up what they know to be a good marriage. No,
they are merely conversing . . . and the words are as weight-
less as air.

Quite apart from the fact that Maud may hear some
of those comments, this sort of judgment tendency, this
babbling on and on must be thoroughly guarded against
by the woman who would be charming. She will carry
over remnants of such a conversation into her next meeting with the victim. She will gradually have a long list of
people upon whom she has sat in horrid judgment, and
toward whom she has a colored opinion that bars her from
easy relationships.

Does this mean you must bury your critical faculties?
Hardly. But you can keep them twice as sharp and efficient
by a different kind of use. Bite down on the day's news
with a vicious appraisal. Read several newspapers with different points of view and get into a violent argument on
the obvious coloring of news. Discuss public personalities
in their public roles. The field is yours, and you can shred

these people to the improvement of your mind, if not the changing of it. Just keep the discussions away from the personal level. Charges of disease, insanity, abnormality,

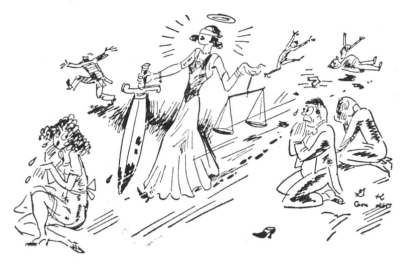

. . . in horrid judgment

and sexual misbehavior may make interesting conversation, but prove nothing. They are usually the refuge of the lazy, gossipy mind.

Why don't you ask?

"I never was so mortified in my life" is the banal start of many a story of great humiliation. It could usually have been avoided by a simple question.

You are asked to go to a dinner party. You've never gone to that house before. It was a phoned invitation, and you are left wondering what to wear. Is it formal, or will an afternoon dress do? This is a time to break with the etiquette books. Don't be lulled by the hour set for dinner. People set their dinner hour for many reasons that have nothing to do with formality. Pick up the phone, call your hostess, and ask her what to wear. If she responds with "Oh, anything, my dear," don't give up. Tell her your dilemma. Shall it be a dinner dress, an evening dress, or an afternoon dress? She'll throw you a lifeline and usually tell you what she is wearing, what her husband is wearing. All the mortification of walking in, dressed out of key with the others, has been avoided.

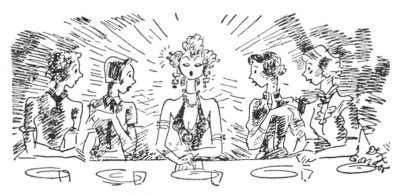

. . . dressed out of key with the others

Remember the spirit of your thank-you's—that we're all just a group of human beings trying to live together. Ask your way along any unfamiliar social situation. Ask the porter what a customary tip is, if you have no idea. Ask the waiter to help you with the foreign language menu. Ask your weekend hostess whether you should tip the maids or merely thank them. If you are to tip, ask what she would recommend as a suitable amount. Ask the guest whose name you didn't hear well to repeat it. Most of all, when you find yourself stranded in a conversation, ask the one who is doing the most informed talking to explain the topic to you. Never be afraid to admit your ignorance if you are interested.

Few of us are so sophisticated that we have met every possible social situation. Almost all of us go through the agonizing moment when it's a matter of bluff and a possible false step. Stop a moment. Have you ever thought anyone a fool because he asked your advice? Of course not. If anything, you respected his wisdom in coming to you. The same psychology applies to this matter of trivial dilemmas. No one will think you gauche when you ask questions. People answer those questions quickly, with a flash of warmth because you turned to them for help. They soon forget the whole matter. It is as childish to stay at sea in a social situation as it is to remain lost in a city where policemen are on every corner to direct you.

Long remember

Remember your introduction to your present "crowd?" The timidity that overcame you just before you went to that first gathering? That awful sense of everyone knowing everyone else, except you? Of conversations going on around you in which you couldn't participate? You do remember? Then remember never to let anyone else go through the same thing without your help and friendliness.

Remember that nightmare you once had of seeing your husband flirt all too seriously with another woman? Your striving for dignity and perspective and your prayer for blindness? You do remember? Then remember never to put another woman through an actual waking nightmare of that sort.

In every group that gets together, from informal bridge parties to gala evening affairs, there will be people going through the same embarrassments that have beset you. If you will exercise your imagination and that much-touted feminine intuition, those people will be easily identified. A little *more* imagination and you will know what to say or do to put the people individually at ease.

Just remember what you wished people had done for you—then do it.

You know why the woman who went to the dressing room twenty minutes ago hasn't returned. She is staying up there because she felt left out. Go get her, casually, as though you merely happened into the room. Bring her back. Bring her into the conversation, or see to it that the men are primed to dance with her. Devote yourself to the inordinately silent man, who is patently shy rather than strong. Discover what he's like, for a highly personal ten minutes. When a friend's husband is obviously drunk, don't pretend all is well. Identify yourself with her by the observation that men are nuisances when they get that way, but with business the strain it is, it's no wonder they do. The man who is flirting violently with you, to the evident discomfiture of his wife—flirt back, but give her a tolerant smile, as though to say, "Aren't they all?"

Last but not least remember that you spend most of your time with women. You are pretty dependent upon their goodwill. The woman who boasts that her friends are all men is headed for social insecurity. She'll get around in her twenties, but she'll sit at home after that, unless she changes her tune. Women are the invitation givers, the social arbiters. Make them your friends, give them your staunchest loyalty. If you don't, you may find yourself practicing allure to the four walls of your own room.

The life of the party

What a maligned phrase it is—"the life of the party." Custom has made it a tag for that most pathetic of creatures, the person who is unsure of himself, and must advertise that fact in an aggressively unpleasant way. The constant talker, the one who always leads some pointless but invariably boisterous prank, the person who guffaws too loudly and too frequently—each one trying to make you recognize his worth. These people are the opposite of the unduly quiet shy person, but they're victims of the same disease—self-consciousness. Pathetic or not, they aren't entertaining. Is it possible to find some simple, always applicable rule that will prevent you from falling into the classification of either the noisy or the silent guest?

Let's go through a dinner party, and see what the common denominator of a pleasant guest would be. You have been invited to a party given for a visiting couple from out of town. You know the date, the hour, the address, and what to wear. And so your preliminary worries are ended. You are going for just two purposes: first, to try to help the visitors enjoy themselves; second, to enjoy yourself. You won't plan any conversations or brood about your approach to these people. You'll have plenty of opportunity to get to know them, their views, their interests, their outlook. The party will be an exciting venture of exploring other people. And that attitude of curiosity and interest is far better popularity ammunition than any rule of thumb about good listening.

And so you arrive at the party. You have come armed with the knowledge that all people are pretty much people. You won't worry about your hair, your powder, your lipstick, the hang of your skirt. You attended to all these at home. You are here to enjoy yourself, and so is everyone else. You acknowledge introductions with a simple, "How do you do, Mrs. Anderson?" Throughout dinner and afterward you are exchanging ideas—talking, listening. If you have time to think of it at all, it dawns on you that you are having a genuinely good time.

The party is over. When you thank your hostess for a pleasant evening, you are being honest. You will be asked back. Anyone who is so sincerely interested in others is invariably asked again.

You will notice that no mention has been made of a dramatic entrance, a brilliant conversation, a sparkling repartee. These are necessary tools for an actress or a playwright, but they have little or nothing to do with charm. The woman who makes herself comfortable with those about her, the woman who makes others feel comfortable with her, will be remembered as delightful after the very witty woman has been dismissed as slightly awe-inspiring.

Use the gifts you have. Use your warmth, your imagination, your kindness; use your wit, too, as long as it is used kindly. The real life of the party is the person who has no time for consciousness of self. She is too busy exploring others, in the friendliest of fashions.

Collectors

There's such a thing as carrying this exploring business too far. Don't bring 'em all back alive. Leave a few. Consider a couple, whom we shall call the Bronsons. He is a sensitive, quiet chap. No one raves about him after he leaves the room, but people remember him as a thoughtful, intelligent man. He is universally courteous and pleasant. He enjoys being with people. But he also enjoys several evenings a week alone with his family. It would be more correct to say he would enjoy those evenings, were he allowed to have them. His wife, alack, is a collector. She has vitality enough to launch a thousand ships with her own two hands. After every party, even the most offhand gathering of friends, she has added at least two names and phone numbers to her encyclopedic directory of "intimates." She takes every "we must see each other sometime" at its face value. And since she's really a pleasant person, those names are glad to accept an invitation the following week.

It isn't her friendliness that should be criticized. She merely lacks discrimination and a sense of proportion. After all, there are just seven days in a week, and her husband works all but one of those days. Yet she admits no limits to her circle of friends. When you are invited for the evening, you will find twice as many people in her apartment as it can comfortably hold, and thrice as many kinds of people as could be congenial. In the face of her husband's protest, she replies with great logic, "Well you seemed to enjoy them a lot over at the Greens'." Her guest

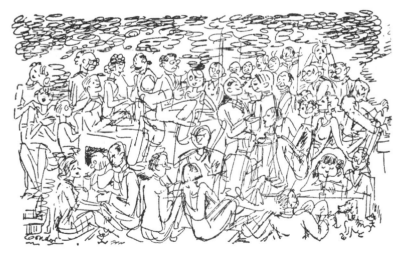

. . . overcrowded free-for-all

list is dwindling and in the wrong direction. Those of her friends whom she likes best are finding a series of excuses not to appear at her house. They refuse to be part of an overcrowded free-for-all, and since they have no way of determining whether they are the important ones to her, they stay away.

The younger version of this collecting instinct is more fortunate. Youngsters like scads of people. They like to go where the whole crowd is gathered. But the wise young hostess varies her program. She reserves an occasional evening when her escort can count on seeing *her,* talking to *her.* Solitaires and sturdy loyalties aren't born in a crowd.

Don't try to collect every interesting or even mildly pleasant person you meet at others' homes. You'll clutter up your life, and so divide yourself that no one gets anything of value from you. Of course, any rule about this is arbitrary, but try to see people once or twice at other parties, after your first meeting, before you invite them to your own.

Scene stealers

The star system is being questioned even in Hollywood. Businessmen are doubting the wisdom of focusing all the action and interest around a single personality. It certainly has no place in our private lives. And don't let your desire to be thought interesting mislead you here. It is not provocative to steal the scene, to have the entire group focusing its attention on you for a long time. The woman who is sure of herself doesn't need this tribute to her prowess.

There is a Mrs. Scene-Stealer in almost every group. She is usually a woman of animation and wit. And in her twenties and thirties she was delightful. Around the bend into her forties, she forgot how to relax. Eternal vigilance became her watchword and scene stealing became a habit. Let's watch her at work. She arrives at a party, always a bit late and usually a bit breathless. She dashes into the living room without taking off her hat and coat (automatically setting herself apart from the rest of us mortals). She has a "telegram"—some vital information or story—for at least three people in the gathering. She can scarcely wait to finish with one person before she must be off to the next, who may be all of two chairs away. Since she is standing, she keeps all the men on their feet. Now that she has all eyes and ears, she launches her general campaign of the newest story, the brightest of repartee. It is only a matter of ten minutes at most before she has the crowd around her. All of this is excellent technique, once. But it goes on evening after evening. The strain begins to show on her face and wear on her friends. She has built a structure on virtuosity rather than on real charm; each evening becomes a major sortie. And at fifty, she's a plain nuisance.

In the younger set there is a Mlle. Scene-Stealer. The boys think she is a wow—for a very short time. They cluster around to listen to her rippling laugh, her flashing words. But in an amazingly short time she finds herself less and less the center of things. She doesn't give any one lad enough chance to shine in his own right. She has bought her audience at the expense of the other girls. Soon she is disliked, dropped, or happily changed into one of the group, taking her fair turn in the limelight.

What is the borderline between being interesting and becoming a nuisance? Good taste, sincerity, and imagination will tell you. If you are late once or twice in your arrival, if you do have something so amusing or so interesting that it can't wait for the removal of your hat and coat, if you have an anecdote that bids fair to put life into an inert group, then you are entitled to the center of the stage. Just as an actress of talent can bring a dying show to life by good timing and good dialogue, so can you. But the actress who steals every scene soon discovers that even the kindest reviews may praise her ability but deplore her show. Your public will avoid your performances, no matter how able, if the rest of the evening seems tepid. They may never lay it to your door, but they know that they seemed like backdrops. And they will avoid the occasion when the backdrop role may be forced upon them.

How to eat in public

No, not which fork or what kind of wine. No one wants to watch you in a restaurant. Barring your host, everyone else would prefer to forget you were there. The smartest atmosphere that can pervade a restaurant is the intangible peace that makes it seem as though each table were in the privacy of its own home. Since it is a communal venture, the only way to achieve that atmosphere is by a certain amount of restraint and thoughtfulness on the part of each diner.

Europeans constantly comment on our abominable restaurant behavior. They seem to have mastered the gentle art of eating in public with more grace than we have. Yet the essence of that art is easily distilled. Modulated voices, patience, consideration for others—these will make us agreeable in restaurants.

The tête-à-tête is quite suitable for café life. You and one other may discuss yourselves and flirt with the greatest aplomb and no one will watch or listen. But the "Did you hear about Nora Smith?" conversation is quite another thing. You know those all-too-frequent luncheons or teas when you and a friend start discussing an absentee. You've heard or overheard these discussions even if you haven't indulged in them. A café seduction can go by almost unnoticed, but just let a name be spoken loud and clear, and watch the eyes turn. From New York City to Albuquerque, there is never a crowd so foreign that the mention of a name won't reach at least one listener who knows your victim. So if you can't keep your voice down (and why can't you?), keep your personalities anonymous.

Your attitude toward the person who serves you, man or woman, is the second revealing feature of eating in public. You have a right to the best service available in the restaurant; notice that word "available." Learn to glance around a restaurant when you come in, get a good idea of how many waiters for how many tables, the length of time it takes to get to the kitchen, the number of people each waiter is taking care of. This isn't difficult. You'll start it as a game, and soon learn to do it in one or two glances. When you've made your estimate, expect service accordingly. And guide your demands as you would in a private home, where you may decide that the maid is incompetent. You certainly don't disturb the other guests because of it.

The waiter is at your mercy and you are at his. He must bear with the humiliation of all manner of personal comments and savage sarcasm. He cannot answer you in the way many attacks should be answered. But he has a neat revenge. He can delay you indefinitely in ways that you can only suspect and never prove. He can be politely aggravating in a series of small irritations. And he can watch your companion writhe at your manners.

After you have summed up the speed you may expect in your chosen restaurant, take a good long look at the face of your waiter. Know him. Ask him any question you choose, about the menu. If you don't know what Eggs Florentine are, ask him. If you are really in a hurry, tell him so, and explain that you realize he is rushed, but could he help you on your way? Treat him as a person who is helping you, not as an ignominious robot. You won't engage him in a long conversation. But you will be able to recognize him, and once he has become a person to you, you will mind your manners.

What can you expect from the waiter? If your food is cold, what should you do? If the meat is tough or not done to your fancy, what should you do? Tell the waiter, of course. But you tell him in the manner of one person telling the agent of another. Remember that he didn't cook the meat. He is the kitchen's delegate to you, and your delegate to the kitchen. Your food will not come back more palatable because you snarled about it. Mistakes in orders, or unsatisfactory dishes are accidents. Do not act as though they were deliberate insults directed at you. Take them calmly, tell your waiter about it as though you knew he would want to know about them, and ask him to correct the mistakes.

Has this any bearing on charm? Ask several dozen people in one large city why they dodge a certain quite important, quite useful young woman in business. Her restaurant behavior is so atrocious that, in a life where much business must be transacted in restaurants, everyone hopes to avoid a public meal with her. Apparently she saves up all the bruises and slights her ego has had for a week or two, and salves them in the restaurant. She has a Roman Emperor complex when dining out.

The experience of dining with her runs something like this. She and her guest or friend go into a restaurant. It is usually a place famous for its celebrities and its aura of scintillating life. By the same token, it is usually crowded, with elaborate menus, tables close together, and busy waiters. Her first sally is a glance around the room, followed by a loud comment on the queer crowd present. Her second is a two-minute debate on which table she'll have, ending in a choice that she accepts as a miserable necessity. Next comes the noisy demand for a menu, and impatient demands for ashtray, water, and "please take away these flowers."

Now comes the survey of the very extensive menu, on which she finds nothing that tempts her. In the same spirit as she accepted her table, she decides to try one or two dishes. But first she asks the waiter for a running description of the ingredients. Her first choice is never her order, because the ingredients never please her. From here on, her poor companion is subjected to a crossfire comment on the people at a nearby table, and criticisms of the food and service. All this is interspersed with very debatable social opinions laid down in the voice of authority. The companion never tries to correct these opinions, or dares suggest disagreement.

If you have dined with this woman or her prototype, you know your role. You only sit and pray that lunch or dinner will soon be over, so that you can slink out as unobtrusively as possible. You may even be guilty of the unfriendly act of catching a stranger's eye to signal that you can't help it.

This girl is pretty. She is well dressed. She is far from stupid. And she could be attractive. But she sits home night after night, alone, and not liking it even a little bit. In a city where much of one's social life is centered in restaurants, no man wants to take her out.

The woman who uses the wrong fork may be engaging; the woman with bad manners toward others never is. So read and remember: the restaurant is just another larger dining room.

The common carrier

If you carry insurance, it probably reads "double indemnity for accidents on common carriers." If you are running a charm score, it should read, "double penalties for offenses

in a common carrier." Busses, trolleys, trains, boats, and
planes are common carriers. And what a multitude of
offenses against graciousness they harbor. You notice we
omit subways, because the crowds prohibit more than
elementary decency and the noise prohibits many of the
usual trespasses.

The chief cause of bad manners in busses and trolleys
is rooted in a strange misconception. Many a woman
who pays a nickel or a dime for her ride expects—nay
demands—the creature comforts she might find in a
Rolls driven by her own chauffeur. Hers is the articulate
attitude that she is used to the finer things of life, including
a seat, "the best people," and privacy. When we say her
attitude is articulate, we mean articulate. She declaims on
the unpleasant people around her, usually with painfully
revealing remarks that have a wide tinge of race prejudice.
If a tired workman beats her to a seat, because he is standing directly in front of it and she is a few feet away, that
brings forth an aristocrat-crack. If someone nudges or
pushes her in the rocky throes of a bus ride, that brings
forth the frozen stare and another comment.

Or she may be the live-and-let-live human who merely
assumes that everyone else on the bus is deaf, and forthwith
regales you with intimate glimpses into her home life; or
amusing anecdotes about newspaper names; or a detailed

but "thoroughly confidential" report on a business matter. Her voice has that odd high pitch that often seems to come with social assurance, but is bad mannered nonetheless.

Man or woman, rich or poor, you have the same status on a common carrier as every other passenger. You have no right to a faraway seat. You are bound by the most rigid rules of courtesy. For crowds, to be bearable at all, must observe a code of tolerance and kindliness that is far broader than smaller group life exacts.

There is only one reason most of us travel. We must get somewhere. Our faces and our bearing upon arrival reflect our traveling experiences. Be rude, allow others to get you distraught, resent those about you, and your face shows all of the scars. Be gracious, accept your companions in common carriers, and your manner reflects serenity.

More than etiquette

No one book on charm can cover all of the manifold aspects of human relations. But we must include a few of the everyday occurrences that make us known for our consideration—or the lack of it.

How are your telephone manners? Keep one picture before you. You may have waited until you had the leisure to call, but you have interrupted the other person without warning. Be brief without being curt. Many people hate to

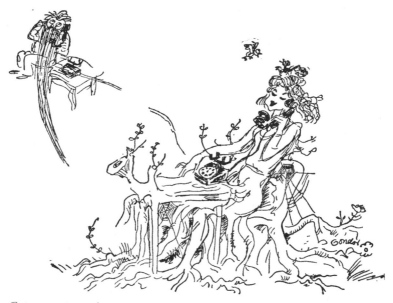

Cut your conversation

talk long on the phone, though they would be lost without it as a useful instrument. Always assume that the other person must be busy, and cut your conversation accordingly.

Are you pleasant on paper? There's a lot of nonsense talked about the art of letter writing. Any literate person can write a gracious letter. Here again, keep one picture in mind. As you start to write, visualize the other person, and talk to him, then write your words down. Write the sort of letter you would like to receive. The only difficult social letter to write is the bread-and-butter note after a visit at which you did not enjoy yourself. The necessity for writing such a letter rarely occurs. When it does, reply briefly but promptly.

Are you one of those women whose friends avoid her on a shopping tour? Then you need to think about two things. First, clarify in your own mind what you want before you go downtown. Second, think about the saleswoman. She stands on her feet all day for a salary that is small compensation for her fatigue. Her salary depends upon completed sales. She receives no credit for selling merchandise which is returned. She must bear with all kinds of customers, all of whom are always right. If you can't decide what you want before you shop, tell her you are only looking. If she has time, she will help you all the more

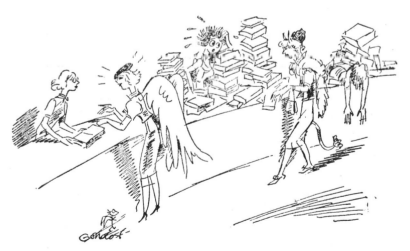

Think about the saleswoman

for your honesty. And don't belittle the merchandise. If it isn't what you want, don't buy. But don't take it out on the saleswoman. She didn't buy it either.

And so we leave this chapter on human relations with one great rule. We're not the first to state it. Try to get inside the skins of others. Think how they feel, how they react, and guide your own conduct by that. It was briefly stated some two thousand years ago. Unfortunately, it is more often quoted than followed. "Do unto others as you would have them do unto you." It's still a sure rule for charm.

6 Realism and Charm

CHARM can't be achieved until you recognize reality—today's situations, today's problems. Frequently these are more decisive factors than the conventions. For these days charm does not necessarily depend upon a strict observation of conventions.

Just a few short years ago, "good women" lived in a walled city. Today's standards are not as clearly demarked. Our very language indicates the change. Profanity on a lady's lips used to be a sign that she was no lady, and perhaps not even a virtuous woman. Profanity today may mean anything from bad taste, or a weak vocabulary, to a superficial talent for doing as the Romans do. A woman working in one of the erstwhile masculine strongholds, such as a newspaper office or a printing house, may find strong language an ever-present help in getting action. The same girl should know that after hours she needs a different set of words for emphasis.

Superficial changes

Fashions in manners change much as fashions in clothes. Indeed, they seem sometimes to take their cue from the clothes. Can you remember the beige meal sack, long-waisted, cut off at the knees, that was the uniform of the nineteen twenties? An abrupt and uncompromising V neck, straight sleeves, and a hideous silhouette, topped off by a *cloche* hat that hid the hair and distorted the face? Can you remember the manner that went with this ugliest of all fashions? We were hard in those days, as brittle and ungraceful as the clothes we wore. We were men among men, cynical, competitive, and our speech and manner reflected our disillusion.

Today that manner is as passé as the costume of the nineteen twenties. It isn't smart to be hard, and we use the word smart in both of its meanings. We have returned to the feminine in dress and attitude. We are not competing with men, but rather working with them. Some of our older sisters, particularly in business, still wear that old chip on their shoulders. Their chins thrust out, their slightest word given drive and emphasis, they march roughshod over ground that has already been broken.

The nineteen thirties and probably the early nineteen forties require a different technique. The successful woman, at home or in business, is the woman who is contributing her efficiency and her talent as a woman. She has invaded the field of architecture because she knows how women like to live in their homes. She has gone into publishing because she knows what women like to read. She has taken over a large part of the advertising world because she knows what to say to make women buy things. Hardness and imitation of men have gone out of fashion.

Mrs. Grundy has died the death in the last twenty years, too. Good and bad, right and wrong, are words that are no longer applied to behavior in simple social situations. Wise and unwise, charming or awkward—these are the gauges by which to measure the multitude of questions that spring from everyday living.

Consider the questions that were so troublesome ten years ago that they were used even in the ads. Should she ask him in? Should a woman visit a man's apartment? Who should write first?

There was a rigid set of rules by which each of these questions could be answered. The trouble with the rules was that most of us couldn't remember them because no reasons, or reasons that we didn't quite accept, were behind the rules. Consider the question about going to a man's apartment. The implications behind the "never" were that the man might attack the woman or that the neighbors spent their evenings watching his front door so that they could "talk." The first implication was an insult to any man you knew well, the second an insult to your own intelligence. But the answer served to keep many a girl who lived in a hall bedroom away from a pleasant evening in a pleasanter room.

Common sense and consideration for others answer every one of those questions to the satisfaction and understanding of a modern woman. Ask anyone in at any hour if you know the person well, and the people around you. It would be foolish to invite a guest into your house if his coming might disturb others who are sleeping, or if the hour is so late that both he and you are weary. It would be awkward to invite him in unless you have a pleasant place in which to entertain him. One crowded bed-living room, after you have dressed in a hurry to go out, is not a pleasant place.

Of course you can invite a man somewhere, after you have given him a mental scrutiny. If he is intelligent, he will appreciate your gracious gesture. But it isn't wise to be overeager and so you would scarcely invite him a second time unless he had reciprocated.

All the way down the list you can answer your own questions. But in all honesty we must remind you of one lingering remnant of our age-old civilization. In man-woman relationships, men still prefer to do the seeking. It might be more cynically phrased that they prefer to think they do the seeking. Here again, apply the yardstick of finesse. Coyness is artificial and silly. In casual social contact, dignity and a mild degree of reserve, added to graciousness, make women attractive to men.

Seriously . . .

There are enough "Courts of Public Opinion," "Counsellors," and "Personal Problems Consultations" so that we would prefer to leave out all discussion of morality and sex in this brief book. Certainly we are not concerned with a long discussion of the right and wrong of affairs, divorces, or other serious relationships between men and women. To offer any advice on sex is, to use a prize-fighting term, leading with your chin. But we called this chapter "Realism and Charm," because there are certain aspects of this question that have a real bearing on charm.

The modern woman is sometimes called upon to decide whether or not to have an affair. It is a fact that "extracurricular" relationships are prevalent. No wonder—in these days when too few men have jobs, fewer have jobs sufficient to support a family, and even those who have jobs are haunted by uncertainty.

Young people live together without bell and book because their joint incomes cannot provide a home. Older people do the same thing for the same reason. Small use to deplore or condemn any of these reasons or results. We are going to discuss the out-of-wedlock relationship solely from the standpoint of charm.

Woman is basically fastidious and possessive. Innate good taste will tell her that the casual affair, bound up with the thought of temporariness, discovery, haste, is not for her. The deeper relationship, the tie between a man and woman who can't get married but who genuinely love each other, is a matter that each person must settle for herself. But no matter what justification, ethically or emotionally, the tie may have, it has a serious count against it in the field of charm.

Affairs are furtive. Affairs at their very best offer no security or permanence. Affairs put a woman on the defensive. She is going against the social code, she has no insurance against ignominious desertion, she must hold her man by constant striving for prettiness, vitality, youth. She has no weapons of custom, public opinion, or usage on her side. When a husband flirts too violently with another woman, a wife can give voice to her objection. The world is with her in her struggle to keep her home in status quo. The mistress must keep silent, never voicing her fear, or speak and give the man the opportunity of reminding her of her fragile hold. The wife can discuss her home problems with other women. She finds help and solace in those discussions that permit her to relax. The mistress, even in a known relationship, will find other women pitted against her. They are quick to condemn her for a breach of taste in admitting the relationship.

This is not to say that men are cads or cruel. But the woman who counts on the "new code," where "marriage is certainly more than a physical thing," and where "you can't make laws about love," must remember one thing. More women than men have accepted that code. We have always accepted deviations from men and have learned to tolerate these deviations. Not so with our average man. Only the exceptional man believes in this "new code."

So, on a morality basis, we have no advice to offer. On the basis of serenity, sureness, and fastidiousness, we recommend the insistence on security and protection that our great-grandmothers were smart enough to demand.

Liquor and ladies

Drinking can be one of the most gracious of modern gestures or one of the most repellent. Turning our eyes away from the hysteria that broke up bars with an ax and looked at liquor from the religious angle, we are considering it entirely from the aspect of harmonious living.

If you do not drink at all, whether from conviction, distaste, or health, you need read only one sentence. IT IS NEVER A MATTER OF DUTY TO DRINK. You can go to the most fashionable cocktail party and still be within the bounds of courtesy in merely saying, "No, thank you," when the drinks are passed. But if you do go to such places, no matter what your reasons for abstinence, avoid any air of disapproval. You need never declare a reason for not drinking. If you are urged to drink, you can reply with, "I really don't care for any," and repeat it as often as a too-insistent host makes necessary. Drinking is not a social asset, like learning to dance well. It is purely a matter of personal preference.

What about consumption of liquor? Would that it were easy to answer. Or that each of us had a little barometer on our wrists that sent up a signal when we had had enough. It doesn't even seem too much to ask that our capacity for the gracious holding of liquor were constant. As it is, one Martini may make us faintly giddy one evening, where three leave us untouched on another occasion. But there are some rather broad rules for drinking, rules that vary with individuals.

The first rule is eat while you drink. From this has grown the canapé custom. Liquor on an empty stomach is quicker in its results than when food is there for it to work upon. So, if you have discovered that you tend to be easily affected by alcohol, go very slowly until after dinner, and not too quickly even then.

The second rule for a quiet stomach, a clear head, and a charming manner is not to mix your drinks. A series of cocktails, wine, gin, and whisky can have only one sequel,

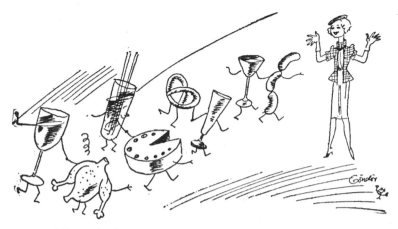

. . . eat while you drink

felt either in the head or the stomach. Better keep to wine if
you start with it, keep to gin drinks, if those were your first
ones, and so on.

The third and most important rule is *stop*. Don't wait
until you get that queer little feeling between the eyes or
that indescribable but always detectable nothing-matters
attitude. If you discover that you are not relaxed and
friendly after a drink or two, make up your mind you probably aren't in the right mood for it, and stop.

We don't say there is no excuse for drunkenness. But
certainly there is no possible hint of charm in that state.
If, by some miscalculation or undue tiredness, you find
yourself in that condition (and stories to the contrary, you'll
know it) make tracks for home as fast as you can. Don't

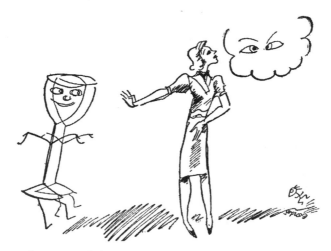

The most important rule is stop

break up a party, don't expect special consideration for your foolishness. Just slip out quickly after being sure you have carfare home, and get there.

It doesn't matter whether you are among friends or strangers, always keep that one little stop signal working, and leave the party if you find yourself feeling befuddled. Let no one detain you. If home is out of the question, stay in the ladies' room until the end of the evening. Never let yourself get so undisciplined that you can't make yourself seek privacy when you need it.

The young girl has her own set of rules for liquor. At the top the list are two words—"Go slow." If you drink at all, nibble food and dance while you make a single drink outlast two or three of your escort's. Alcohol permits your elders to feel young and carefree again. But you don't need it. It will not help your figure, your skin, or your eyes. Indeed it tends to do the opposite. So go slow. And never feel that you are a goody-good if you don't drink at all.

As frequent as the personal problem of how much to drink is the lady's dilemma of what to do with an escort who followed no rules at all. Circumstances change the answer so often that we can give only one guide. No matter

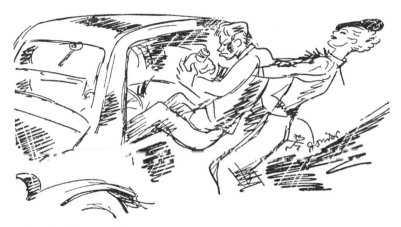

Do not let him go off alone . . .

what other things you find necessary to bear with, don't let him drive a car. Plead with him, reason with him, knock him out, or call a policeman. But neither ride with him nor let him go off alone driving a car while drunk.

Before that final decision, when you are still partying with him, are there any laws of charm that function? Yes, no matter how irritated you may be with him, remember he didn't set out to be unpleasant. Try to regard the incident as you would if he were taken unexpectedly ill. Unless you have the misfortune to be married to him, you don't need to repeat the experience, unless you find that his sober qualities far outweigh his cuppish tendencies.

The poor dear

There may have been a time when the poor dear had her place. She was the martyr. She was the wife who slaved, the woman who enjoyed poor health, the woman who played bridge though she hated it, the woman who gave her life to her children or her parents or her relatives. She did whatever was suggested to her as being noble and fine. And that was that. Or rather, that was only the beginning. She made all innocent bystanders a party to her self-sacrifice.

Conversational or social self-sacrifice has gone out. The poor dear is rightly regarded as a bore and a fraud today. You are not expected to make any sacrifices that cost so dearly that you must be paid in eternal gratitude. You are not supposed to give up anything voluntarily unless you can do it without referring to it again. And if all that sounds selfish and callous, it is really quite the contrary. The martyr always advertises her nobility and is the most difficult of egotists.

Let's see how this greater honesty works out in everyday situations. Should you offer to ride in the rumble seat when wind and cold bring on real distress? By no means. It is just as gracious to say, "I'd like to be the one to suffer back there, but you would suffer later, if I did, so someone else will have to rumble." When it's a question of light or dark

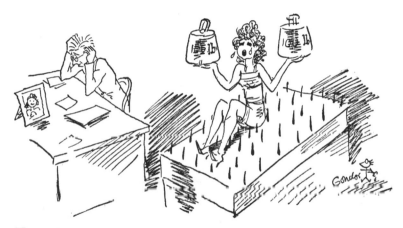

The martyr . . .

meat and you are asked your choice, you are supposed to admit your preference. The perpetual wing-eater has gone out of fashion. When there are five people and bridge is the game at hand, take your turn cutting in and out. Don't martyr yourself by staying out of the game. You're bound to mention it later or expect special treatment for your sacrifice, if you do. Be quick to say what movie you have seen, what show you don't want to see, what your choice of an evening's entertainment is. You may be over-ruled and you'll accept that with good grace. But go on record. Silent suffering is a nasty form of vanity.

Establish a reputation for being predictable. Let people know what you want and like. Do it graciously. People like the woman with whom they are comfortable, and the wishy-washy poor dear is a burden both to herself and others.

Money matters

It must have been much easier to be a gracious woman in those periods of history when we were supposed to be helpless and utterly unaware of the facts of life, particularly the sordid money facts. The girl at home demanded of her family all she could think to ask for, sulked over the refusals, and cheated her way around the extravagances that couldn't be explained. Matrons went through many of the same devices with their husbands. They were aware of money, but as something that depended upon the moods of their menfolk rather than the world outside. A lot of this attitude still hangs over. We know more than one married woman who fibs about the price of a new dress, and lives in dread of the day the charge account bill comes in the mail.

Women are still not very realistic about money. Too few of them work for it to understand how to manage it. Managing money here does not mean saving it. It means the judicious *use* of money. And so it is no wonder we are occasionally lacking even in basic honesty in the matter of dollars and cents.

Consider the woman shopper. How many of your friends have told you, with no sense of shame, about the merchandise they have bought, used, and returned? Any clerk in a store can give you instance after instance of the evening dress that has been worn and then credited back. Quite apart from morals, the picture of a woman who wants to be lovely yet lies and cheats for the sake of a new dress, is incongruous. Distinction is built on a sounder foundation than mere appearance. It cannot rest on a basis of childishness. We don't say you never should buy what you can't afford, even though you do manage to pay for it. But we do say that you should not buy, wear, and then return merchandise, unless that merchandise is truly faulty. That is rank dishonesty and the cause of higher prices in stores.

The woman downtown in general is frequently unattractive in money matters. Watch her with a friend at a restaurant, arguing about who is to pay the bill. Watch her debate with herself about tips. Watch her hold up a whole ticket window line while she argues for $1.65 seats. She has learned neither to departmentalize her pocketbook, nor to make her financial arrangements beforehand. When she has had more experience with money, she will know how to arrange with her friend who is to be guest and who hostess. She will know that a 10 percent tip is standard, except when

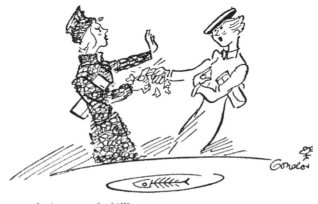

. . . who is to pay the bill?

that tip figures to less than a dime or when the service has been unusually good. She will arrange for her theatre tickets beforehand or be prepared to spend the extra amount her negligence has cost her. And her life will run smoothly, with none of those ghastly lulls when she is doing sums in her head or fumbling in her handbag.

But when one speaks of charm, or when one wants to acquire it, it is usually because there is a gentleman in the offing. One of the hardest barriers to complete naturalness in casual social life between men and women is the money question. Should you let a young man take you to the theatre in $1.10 seats or would he value you more if you dressed for the orchestra? Does he fail to bring you flowers because he is stingy, thoughtless, or impoverished? When he asks you where you want to go, should you name a tearoom or a supper club? When he asks you what you want for a gift, should you say "Nothing" or "Guerlain perfume"? How on earth are you supposed to know what the man can spend on you? How can you steer a middle course between being a gold digger and a church mouse?

One of the most popular young women we know has solved this dilemma in the most effortless manner. She takes nothing for granted. She doesn't try to judge the man's financial status by his clothes, car, or job. She goes out with poor young men and sons of great wealth, with equal ease and adaptability. She is apt to be seen in a newspaperman's grill on Second Avenue one night and at the Waldorf the next. Her secret? She asks the man what he can afford! And she does it in the friendliest manner. When he asks her what she would like to do, she counters with, "Want to make it a $3 evening or a 'bust'?" She can do it. So can you. All it takes is a security within yourself, a feeling of friendliness toward your escort.

You don't need to have money spent on you as a token of prestige. Money should be merely the boundary line of an evening. Within whatever boundary the man mentions, you will enjoy yourself. But one word of caution and advice here. Read your local papers, talk to your friends, and keep your ears open, so that you can suggest types of places within different budgets. Almost every large city has some sort of magazine that describes its entertainment. Familiarize yourself with it. And this holds true even if it is a husband and not a swain who suggests an evening of entertainment.

With one last word about money, we'll drop the subject, only advising you to face money facts honestly. Don't be afraid to borrow money, if it is a life and death matter. Don't be afraid to borrow money that you know the lender can spare and that you can return within the time you mention. But don't be angry if you are refused. And don't hesitate to refuse to lend if you can't afford it. Credit is a normal part of our everyday life. But it isn't a matter of friendship. Leave charm at the door and go as a businesswoman.

Face the facts

They used to call it change of life—those difficult forties and fifties when women become problems to their families and friends. We don't question the physiology involved. But we do know that much of the trouble inherent in these years has its roots in ways of thought and attitudes way back in the early nineteen twenties and mid-thirties.

If one short sentence could be read and learned and felt by all women, there would be fewer neurotic women wandering around. LEARN TO LIVE WITH YOURSELF. Make yourself over as much as is necessary to adapt your life to others, but accept yourself as you really *are*. If you are a worldling who loves bright lights and fleshpots, you may well have to do without them, but always know that the denial is not changing your inherent yen. If you are a quarrelsome individualist, modify and restrain yourself for social reasons, but admit to yourself that you are essentially quarrelsome.

You need no apologies for yourself, though you may need some for bad conduct. One of the most miserable women of our acquaintance is a housewife who has been a very good housewife though she started out as a sculptress. She has never been able to accept herself as a frau. Her pseudo-frustration in art has made a completely nasty human being of her. One of the most virtuous ladies who is inherently a pagan has become the meanest and narrowest of Puritans in middle life, eager to condemn all others who have had the very things she hankered for so secretly. And one of the easiest, happiest, and most amiable females of our circle is one who blithely admits she is unreasonable, inclined to be querulous, and frankly greedy. Not that she acts all these things, but when she does occasionally act any one of the three, she doesn't dress it up in any fancy dress.

When you find yourself getting jittery and irritable, face the facts. Find out why. It isn't because people are abusing you. It's because you are whatever you are. Get in the habit of calling yourself honest if ugly names. Is your husband too flirtatious, or are you possessive and none too sure of yourself? Are you overworked, or are you rather incompetent? It will do you and your exterior no real harm when you find yourself getting green with envy over Mrs. Jones's better fortune—as long as you admit to yourself that you are greedy and envious.

Our true faults do not distort and spoil us. Our refusal to admit them, to accept ourselves as very inadequate human beings, is ruinous. So get rid of your need to think of yourself as a heroine. Know every one of your mean, petty, unreasonable traits. Then learn either to get rid of them or to live with them. And it is just possible that you may erase those qualities that make the record look too unpleasant. But, best of all, you won't need to justify yourself to yourself by all the unpleasant devices so common to women today.

No one else need know your honest names for yourself. Indeed it is far better not to go in for confessionals to friends. But don't be afraid to admit your follies to yourself.

Fact-facing means an honest self-admission of age. The woman of fifty can be vivacious, attractive, enchanting—

but only if she knows she is fifty. Let her struggle for the attributes of thirty, and she is ridiculous. Let her assume the privileges of seventy, and she is pathetically ancient before her time.

Does this have a relation to charm? How agreeable is the woman who is always telling you how much she puts up with in her home life? How can she be compared to the woman who tells you nothing because she knows she is unreasonable, nagging, demanding? How fascinating is the woman who tells you about the slights she has suffered at the hands of the club ladies? How does she compare with the woman who knows she doesn't seem to inspire club confidence, and so keeps quiet? Which woman would you describe as judicious—the one who mentions a neighbor's new car as another ostentatious gesture which the neighbor could ill afford, or the woman who says nothing, knowing she is jealous and might show it?

Charm is much like a beautiful dress. It can be acquired. But it means very little unless the personality it covers is clean and properly cared for.

Charming people

Can you learn to charm people? Can you learn how to go forth and cast a spell over friends and acquaintances? Can you acquire a few easy tricks that give you this sorcery?

If you bought this book hoping to acquire an *abracadabra* or *open sesame*—a new version of three easy lessons—you certainly know it isn't our philosophy. If charm could be reduced to devices, there would be no disagreeable people left.

But you are well on your way when you admit you wish to be liked. You've gone that first step of admitting that you want esteem, prestige, popularity. In short, you've been honest. The rest of the way is just a reversal of the picture. You must recognize that what you want, others want, too. Give others esteem, prestige, warmth, friendliness, and you will be living with charming people.

It isn't done with trickery. It's done by getting rid of guile and brittle wisdom. It's done by going back to the simple friendly approach of your childhood, when all you needed to remember was to be kind, because you were already completely unafraid.

People talk about the charm of childhood, as though it were a matter of age. It isn't. The vital essence of childish unself-consciousness can permeate your personality through life. It removes fear. It stirs a perennial curiosity about the world and the people in it. It generates so lively an interest in other people that it overcomes narrow preoccupation with self.

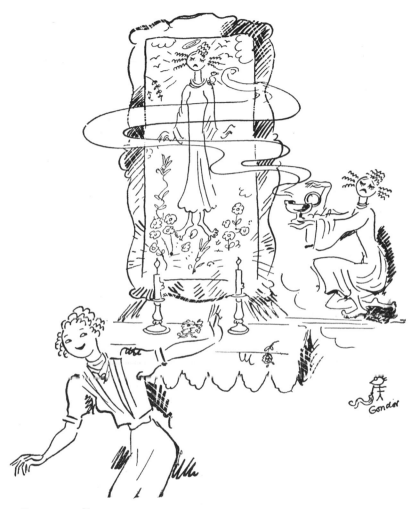

Forget yourself

When you meet people in a spirit of friendly, confident interest, sure that they are flesh and blood and kin to you, they will find you gracious. Add kindness, the quick word or gesture of reassurance when they falter—and they will find you devastating. This is no formula. It is a real change of heart, a switching of interest from yourself to others. And it casts that spell called charm. All the rest—the beauty aids, the clothes, the fastidiousness, the well-dressed figure, the active mind—are necessary. They let you forget yourself and think of others as only a sure person can. But they are mere stage sets for a show that is bound to fail unless you forget to be a star and remember that you are one with your public.

APPENDIX

A Caloric Table of Everyday Foods*

Food	100 Calories
Almonds, salted	10–12 nuts
Apple, baked with sugar	½ apple
Apple dumpling	⅓ medium dumpling
Apple, fresh	1 large apple
Apple pie	piece 1½ inches at circumference
Apple sauce	⅜ cup
Apricots, dried, stewed, sweetened	¼ cup
Asparagus, canned	15 large stalks 5½ inches long
Asparagus, fresh	20 large stalks 8 inches long
Asparagus soup, cream of	½ cup (scant)
Bacon	4–5 small slices
Baking powder biscuit	2 small biscuits
Bananas	1 medium
Beans, baked, canned	⅓ cup
Beans, lima, fresh or canned	½ cup
Bean soup	¾ cup
Beans, string	2⅓ cups of 1-inch pieces
Beef, broth	2½ cups
Beef, corned, boiled (with fat)	slice 4½ inches by 1½ inches by 1¼ inches
Beef, dried	4 thin slices 4 inches by 5 inches
Beef, Hamburg steak, broiled	cake 2½ inches diameter, ⅞ inch thick
Beef liver, broiled, ground	½ cup
Beef, loaf	slice 4 inches by 6 inches by ⅛ inch
rib, lean, roasted	slice 5 inches by 2½ inches by ¼ inch
round, lean, pot roast	slice 4¾ inches by 3½ inches by ⅛ inch
sirloin steak, lean, broiled	slice 2 inches by 1½ inches by ¾ inch
stew with vegetables	⅖ cup
Beets, fresh	4 beets, 2 inches diameter (1⅓ cups sliced)
Blackberries, fresh	½ cup (50 berries)
Bologna sausage	slice 2⅛ inches diameter, ½ inch thick
Bran muffins	1 small muffin

*These tables are quoted from *Overweight and Underweight,* a pamphlet issued by The Metropolitan Life Insurance Company, and adapted from *A Laboratory Handbook for Dietetics,* by Mary Swartz Rose, The Macmillan Company, New York, 1929. They are reproduced here by permission of the author and The Macmillan Company.

Food	*100 Calories*
Bran, prepared	½ cup
Brazil nuts, shelled	2 nuts
Bread, white, medium loaf	slice ½ inch thick
toast, medium loaf	slice ½ inch thick
graham, medium loaf	slice ½ inch thick
whole wheat, medium loaf	slice ½ inch thick
Bread pudding	1 level tablespoon
Broccoli	2⅓ cups
Brown Betty	⅕ cup
Butter	1 tablespoon or 1 square 1¼ inches by 1¼ inches by ¼ inch
Buttermilk	1⅛ cups
Cabbage	3½ cups chopped (4–5 cups shredded)
Cake, chocolate layer	½ small slice
coffee	1½ inch cube
Cantaloupe	1 melon 4½ inches diameter
Carrots, fresh	1⅔ cups of ½ inch cubes (4–5 young carrots 3–4 inches long)
Cauliflower	1 small head 4½ inches diameter
Celery	4 cups of ¼ inch pieces
Celery soup, cream of	½ cup
Charlotte Russe	½ serving
Cheese, American	1⅛ inch cube
Camembert	⅘ of 1 sector
Roquefort	piece 1½ inches by 1¼ inches by ⅞ inch
soft cream	2 tablespoons
soufflé	½ cup
Swiss	slice 4½ inches by 3½ inches by ⅛ inch
Cheese straws	3 straws 5 inches by ⅜ inch by ⅜ inch
Cherries, sweet, fresh	20 cherries
Chicken, lean meat, cooked	3 slices 3½ inches by 2½ inches by ¼ inch
roast	1 slice 4 inches by 2½ inches by ¼ inch
salad	¼ cup
Chocolate, beverage made with milk	½ cup (scant)
blanc mange	¼ cup (scant)
fudge piece	1½ inches by ¾ inch by 1 inch
layer cake	½ small slice
nut caramels	piece 1 inch by 1 inch by ⅘ inch
Clam chowder	¾ cup

Food	*100 Calories*
Clams	12 clams or ⅔ cup
Cocoa, beverage, with milk & water, half-and-half	⅔ cup
Codfish, creamed	½ cup
Cod-liver oil	1 tablespoon
Coleslaw	1 cup
Consommé	4 cups
Cookies, plain	2 cookies 2¼ inches diameter
Corn bread	slice 2 inches by 2 inches by 1 inch
Corn, canned	⅓ cup
chowder	⅓ cup
fresh, on cob	2 ears 6 inches long
soup, cream of	½ cup
Cornflakes	¾ cup
Cornmeal, cooked	⅔ cup
Cornstarch blanc mange	¼ cup
Cottage pudding	slice 1¾ inches by 2 inches by 2½ inches
Crab meat, canned	¾ cup
Crackers, graham	2½ crackers 2½ inches by 2¾ inches
oyster	24 crackers 1 inch in diameter
rye	5 crackers 1¾ inches by 3½ inches
saltines	6 crackers 2 inches square
soda	4 crackers 2¾ inches by 2½ inches
whole wheat	4½ crackers 2½ inches by 1¾ inches
Cranberry sauce	¼ cup (scant)
Cream, thick (40 percent fat)	1⅔ tablespoons
thin (18.5 percent fat)	¼ cup (scant)
Cream filling (custard)	3⅓ tablespoons
Cucumbers	2 cucumbers 9 inches long
Cup custard	⅓ cup
Custard, boiled	⅓ cup (scant)
Custard pie	piece 2 inches at circumference
Dates, unstoned	3–4 dates
Doughnuts	½ doughnut
Egg	1 large (average size 70 calories)
Escarole	2 large heads
Farina	¾ cup
Figs, dried	1½ large
Floating island	2 tablespoons (heaping)
Frankfurters	1 sausage

Food	100 Calories
French dressing with salad oil	1½ tablespoons
Fruitcake	piece 1⅞ inches by 1⅞ inches by ⅜ inch
Fruit cocktail	⅜ cup
Fruit salad	¼ cup and ½ tablespoon dressing
Ginger ale	1½ cups
Gingerbread, sour milk	piece 1 inch by 2 inches by 2 inches
Gingersnaps	6 snaps 1¾ inches diameter
Grapefruit	½ large
juice	1⅓ cups
Grape juice	½ cup
Grapes, Malaga	20–25 grapes
Griddle cakes	1 cake 4½ inches diameter
Halibut steak	piece 3 inches by 1¼ inches by 1 inch
Ham, boiled	slice 4¾ inches by 4 inches by ⅛ inch
Hard sauce	1 tablespoon
Hash	¼ cup (scant)
Hominy grits, cooked	⅘ cup
Honey	1 tablespoon
Ice cream, commercial	¼ cup
Jellies	approximately 1 tablespoon
Lady fingers	2–4 fingers
Lamb chops, broiled	lean meat of one chop 2 inches by 1½ inches by ¾ inch
Lamb, leg, roast	slice, 3½ inches by 4½ inches by ⅛ inch
Lemon ice	½ cup (scant)
Lemon jelly	½ cup
Lemon juice	1⅛ cups
Lemon meringue pie	piece 1 inch at circumference
Lettuce	2 large heads
Macaroni and cheese	½ cup
Macaroons	2 macaroons
Mackerel, Spanish, broiled	cross-section 2½ inches on back
Maple syrup	1½ tablespoons
Marshmallows	5 marshmallows 1¼ inches diameter
Mayonnaise dressing	1 tablespoon
Milk, condensed, sweetened	1½ tablespoons
dried, whole	3 tablespoons (scant)
evaporated	3¾ tablespoons
skim	1⅛ cups
whole	⅝ cup

Food	*100 Calories*
Mince pie	piece 1 inch at circumference
Mints, chocolate cream	3 mints 1 inch diameter
Molasses	1½ tablespoons
Molasses cookies	3 cookies 2 inches diameter
Muffins	¾ muffin
Mushrooms, fresh	20–25 mushrooms 1 inch diameter
Oats, rolled, cooked	½ to ¾ cup
Oleomargarine	1 tablespoon
Olive oil	1 tablespoon
Olives, green or ripe	6–8 olives
Onions	3–4 medium
creamed	⅓ cup
Orange juice	1 cup
Oranges	1 large
Oyster stew	¾ cup
Oysters	⅔ cup solids or 6–15 oysters, depending on size
Parsnips	1 parsnip 7 inches long, 2 inches diameter
Peaches, canned	2 large halves and 3 tablespoons juice
fresh	3 medium
stewed	½ cup
Peanut brittle	2 squares 1¼ inches by 1¼ inches by ⅜ inch
Peanut butter	1 tablespoon (scant)
Peanuts	20–24 single nuts
Pears, canned	3 halves and 3 tablespoons juice
fresh	2 medium
Peas, canned	¾ cup
creamed	½ cup
green, shelled	¾ cup
Pea soup, green, cream of	⅔ cup
Pea soup, split	⅗ cup
Pecans, shelled	12 meats
Peppers, green	5 peppers 3½ inches long
stuffed	1 large
Pineapple, canned	1 slice and 3 tablespoons juice, or ¼ cup, shredded
fresh	2 slices 1 inch thick
juice	⅔ cup
Plums, fresh	3–4 large
Popovers	1 popover
Pork chops, broiled	½ average chop (lean meat only)
Pork sausage, cooked	1⅔ sausages 3 inches long, ¾ inch diameter